CONTENTS

KV-638-590

CHANGING MINDS

OUR LIVES AND MENTAL ILLNESS

CHANGING MINDS

OUR LIVES AND MENTAL ILLNESS

**Edited by Rosalind Ramsay, Anne Page,
Tricia Goodman and Deborah Hart**

GASKELL, LONDON

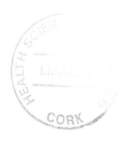

British Library Cataloguing-in-Publication Data
A catalogue record for this book is available from the British Library.
ISBN 1-901242-88-9

The Royal College of Psychiatrists is a registered charity (no. 228636).

Printed in the UK by Henry Ling Limited, at the Dorset Press, Dorchester DT1 1HD.

Cover picture: *Hospital Ward (Banstead Hospital)* by Rosemary Carson (36" x 24", oil on board).

CONTRIBUTORS

Susan Bailey	Consultant Psychiatrist, Salford NHS Trust
David Baldwin	Honorary Consultant Psychiatrist, West Hampshire NHS Trust
Jamie Barnes	Cumbria
Susan Benbow	Consultant Psychiatrist, Manchester Mental Health Partnership
Kam Bhui	Consultant Psychiatrist, South London and Maudsley NHS Trust
Steve Bloomfield	Media and Information Manager, Eating Disorders Association
Jim Bolton	Consultant Psychiatrist, South West London and St George's NHS Trust
Peter Byrne	Consultant Psychiatrist, St Patricks Hospital, Dublin
Alison Cobb	Policy Officer, Mind, London
Michael Crowe	Consultant Psychiatrist, South London and Maudsley NHS Trust
Nicola Dacre	Portsmouth
Stephen Dominic	Address supplied
Colin Edington	County Durham
Roger Farmer	Consultant Psychiatrist, Kingston and District Community NHS Trust
Daisy Fields	Address supplied
Emily Finch	Consultant Psychiatrist, South London and Maudsley NHS Trust
Roger Freeman	Former Consultant Psychiatrist, Hillingdon Hospital NHS Trust
Lizzie Gardiner	London
Tricia Goodman	Team Leader, West London Health Promotion Agency
Alison Gray	Consultant Psychiatrist, Worcestershire Community Healthcare NHS Trust
Peter Grist	Surrey
Deborah Hart	Head of External Affairs, Royal College of Psychiatrists
Gillian Harrison	London
Mike Hobbs	Consultant Psychiatrist, Oxfordshire Mental Healthcare NHS Trust
Philip Ingram	Suffolk
Jean James	Gwent
Michael King	Professor of Psychiatry, Royal Free Hampstead NHS Trust
Barry Lane	Spain
Isaac Marks	Emeritus Professor, South London and Maudsley NHS Trust
Kay McKall	Ipswich
Winston McCartney	Northern Ireland Association for Mental Health
Keith Murray	Address supplied
V. I. Oliver	London

Adamson Collection

A collection of 40 000 paintings, drawings, sculptures and ceramics produced by patients who worked with the pioneering art therapist Edward Adamson from 1946 to the mid-1990s. The collection is housed and displayed by the South London and Maudsley NHS Trust and is under the curatorship of Alice Jackson, Reay House, 108 Landor Road, London SW9 9NT (tel: 020 7411 6371). The works published in this book are all anonymised.

Acknowledgements

The Editors thank the West London Health Promotion Agency for their advice and generous financial support, and the Henry Boxer Gallery, London (www.henryboxergallery.com) for supplying the cover image, reproduced by kind permission of the artist, Rosemary Carson.

FOREWORD

This is an unusual book. It is full of honest comments and telling observations within what is often a taboo arena. It invites one to 'stop, think, and understand'– one of the punch lines of the current Royal College of Psychiatrists' five year long campaign to combat the stigmatisations and discriminations against people with mental illnesses. I consider the awkward pluralisation of these words to be important in reminding us of the variety of prejudices and their origins that colour our attitudes and behaviour in this matter.

Nature, in the interests of species survival, has always led us over-inclusively to label as negative and then sometimes irrationally confront or avoid those we find or expect to be 'different' from us. As if that is not enough inherent potential prejudice, the human psyche can be so personally fragile that we even more fearfully defend against any perceived distressing differences in emotional expression and related behaviour in others. Thus, if personally vulnerable in this way, then encountering those with mental illnesses may threaten the breakdown of our own defences, promoting our further condemnations of, distancing from and discriminations against them. All this occurs, both surprisingly and unsurprisingly, while as many as one in four of us can expect to experience serious mental health problems, often amounting to a mental illness, at some time in our own lives.

These reports indeed serve to remind us how different the mental illnesses are, the one from the other. Misperceived 'dangerousness' can fuel the isolation of those with some disorders; patronising and personally reassuring condemnation of others on the grounds of their 'self-infliction' can reduce self-esteem even further and stifle their struggle to recover. The distancing that comes from convictions that all people with mental illness are impossible to communicate or empathise with inevitably renders all those afflicted as even more 'unpredictable'. People with many illnesses can develop inevitable social handicaps. When the illness is 'physical', compassion and public assistance are commonplace; not so with mental illnesses.

Psychiatry is often condemned for attaching labels to mental health problems. Such labels can carry the hazard, for the individual concerned, of him or her being thereafter permanently and readily stigmatised and then discriminated against. Such labels can be justified and invaluable only if they both permit the sufferer to have his or her separate identity respected for what it is; and also enable logical, managed and focused treatment to make a real and beneficial difference to outcome. This is the essence of good medical practice and is the route that psychiatrists, as medical practitioners, can often justify and must expect to be required to do so at all times.

Meanwhile, psychiatrists and other caring groups and institutions must search for their common ground as well as their differences if the interests of those of us afflicted with one or other mental illness are to be served. We should remember that biological diversity and cultural diversity, if accompanied by mutual respect, can maximise human development.

The College's current anti-stigma campaign, now entering its fifth year, is open to inspection, both of its toolkit (being developed to empower one and all) and its projects (twenty or more in number, either launched or in the making). These ingredients of the campaign can be explored through the developing campaign website (http://www.rcpsych.ac.uk/campaigns/cminds/index.htm) and otherwise by contacting the campaign office at the College, 020 7235 2351 ext. 122.

I greatly value the opportunity to write this brief preface to such an important addition to our toolkit at this stage.

Professor Arthur Crisp
Chairman
Campaign Management Committee
Changing Minds

PREFACE

Recognition of the needs of people with mental health difficulties is growing. We are becoming more aware of the stigma and discrimination people may face because of their problems. Stigma has a harmful effect on people's everyday lives, their relationships, work and so on. This has led to a number of initiatives to increase the public's understanding of mental illness and to fight the stigma attached to it. This book is one part of the Royal College of Psychiatrists' 'Changing Minds: Every Family in the Land' anti-stigma campaign.

In 1999 the Royal College of Psychiatrists and West London Health Promotion Agency joined forces to produce a book that would create the chance for individuals to tell their own stories. The final collection is much richer than we could ever have imagined when we began. You will read here about doctors who are patients and patients who are employed as mental health workers, about psychiatrists who question the way they work, voluntary organisations that strive to improve services and repeatedly of individuals who have discovered ways to make sense of events that seemed hard to understand and beyond their control at the time. You will also read about the experiences of people who live with someone with a mental illness.

We hope these stories will speak for themselves about the impact of mental health problems on individuals and their friends and family. They describe the diversity of experience. Some of the stories are negative, others more hopeful in outlook, but all look at how people learn different ways to get on with their lives. We recognise that putting thoughts about one's experiences into words can be cathartic. We also recognise the courage of people who have been able to be so open in talking about themselves. On request some authors have used a pseudonym.

We have included commentaries with the stories, not to suggest the authors have any answers, but to try and widen the discussion.

We believe that people dealing with similar problems may gain some hope from knowing about possible ways forward, and carers and professionals too will appreciate the real inside knowledge shared here.

Our thanks go to all the contributors, and to anyone who helped to put us in contact with them. We thank the Publications Department at the Royal College of Psychiatrists and the West London Health Promotion Agency for backing the project. We also thank organisations supporting the Royal College of Psychiatrists' 'Changing Minds: Every Family in the Land' anti-stigma campaign: the Department of Health, Mind and the College Membership.

Rosalind Ramsay, Anne Page, Tricia Goodman and Deborah Hart

STIGMA

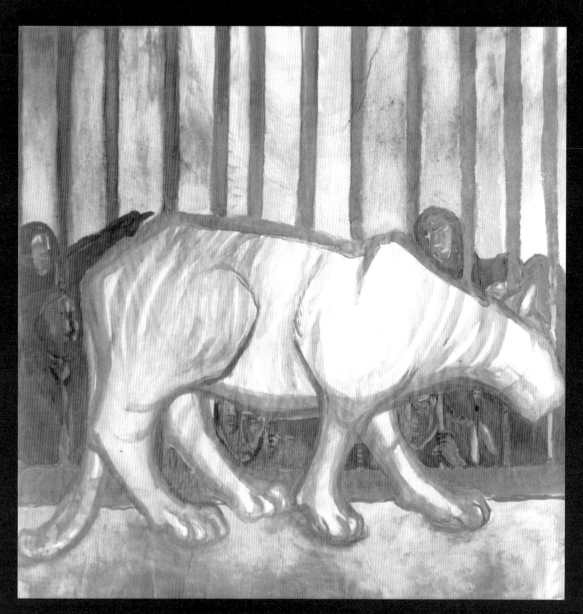

From the Adamson Collection

What happens when a black hole opens in our lives? We can't get on and do things. The best that seems possible is for there to be someone available to listen to how we feel and to understand how overwhelmingly incapacitating it is to have severe depression.

This is how a day with severe depression feels like to me.

It's hard to say when one day ends and the next one starts, as it feels as if it is a never ending struggle to get through the next twenty-four hours. After the endless battle of trying to survive, when all you can feel and see is another uphill struggle, the only way you know the difference in time is lightness and darkness; when it's light you know it must be day and when it's dark it has to be night. Why can't life be as simple?

When you try to unwind at the end of the day you drag yourself to bed. Then what happens? The mind decides it's time to go into overdrive and to have a journey all of its own and you follow it back in time, as if caught in a time warp going over events from childhood; some good times, some not so good. It's funny how life always brings the bad and negative thoughts back to you with more detail, and the happy times just come and go in a flash. You're so frustrated you can't get to sleep no matter how hard you try, so you decide to get up out of bed for a drink, and go back to bed hoping to get some sleep, thinking you will have a better day tomorrow.

A day with severe depression

Colin Edington

It's easy to hide behind a plastic smile, even easier to walk across to the other side of the road. That way friends can't ask, 'How are you?' You may turn to say, 'Oh, I'm fine,' but sometimes you feel like screaming 'I feel bloody terrible.' What will they say, 'Pull yourself together…' This is the last thing you want to hear, if you are able to do just that you would have done so.

You keep saying people don't understand how vulnerable you feel, and that they should realise that it is an illness you are suffering from. 'I wish we could change places for just one day, so that you can see and experience what it is like.' Maybe then people will be able to treat sufferers with compassion and make us feel that we do not have to hide our feelings, or be subject to the stigma and remarks made out of ignorance and fear of mental health problems. After all, mental illness does not have any age limits or class barriers and may affect anyone at sometime during their life. People ask what it is like to have a depressive illness. It's hard to explain how even the simplest of everyday tasks becomes very difficult.

Some of the worst times are when you are really down because your concentration takes a holiday. If someone is not there to check on you anything may happen. When you have a high it can be a frightening time as you are aware that once the high subsides you will end up feeling even lower and more depressed. While you are having a high the feeling is brilliant, but it doesn't last very long.

It can't be normal depending on drugs to live a normal life.

There is the highlight of your month or whenever you see your consultant psychiatrist and you tell him how you have been since the last visit. It's always good to talk to someone who knows or understands the problems and fears of depression; at least we hope so?

Because of the illness you feel so vulnerable, and you don't want to let anyone get close to you, as you feel you always lose those closest to you. You are sceptical of people and feel that it's hard to trust them with your emotions.

When you try and have a night out and forget about the depression, as soon as you walk into a club you feel as if every eye in the building is looking through you. You feel isolated, as if the walls are closing in, and you just have to escape – so you end up having no social life at all.

When the nights get longer, this is the worst time of year as you feel as if you are a prisoner in your own home.

COMMENTARY – PETER RELTON

'I wrote *The Loony-bin Trip* between 1982 and 1985. Now, when I reread it, I find something in it rings false… typing it over I want to say, Wait a moment – why call this depression? – why not call it grief? You've permitted your grief, even your outrage, to be converted into a disease.' Kate Millett (1991)

Many people in the mental health field, professionals and users alike, want to combat the stigma experienced by people with a 'mental illness' by promoting the idea that mental illnesses are just like other diseases. Those with mental illness, the argument goes, should no more be blamed for their affliction than someone with cancer should be blamed for having cancer.

Colin's account accepts this view: 'You keep saying people don't understand how vulnerable you feel, and that they should realise that it is an illness you are suffering from.'

Yet problems arise when our distress is pathologised as a disease.

When someone is given a mental illness label, the problem is focused within the individual rather than looking at the social context of a person's life experiences. Emphasis is placed on medical treatment – drugs or even electroconvulsive therapy (ECT). I am not denying that drugs are effective for some people, some of the time (particularly for short periods). But there is a blanket assumption, shared by the general public as well as by many mental health professionals, that drugs are necessary long-term for everyone with a particular diagnosis. And I find this worrying.

Here is another comment made by the writer:

'It can't be normal depending on drugs to live a normal life.'

A mental illness diagnosis in itself brings with it a profound sense of failure and of being different from (i.e. inferior to) everybody else. Long-term reliance on medication reinforces this sense of inferiority and failure. Other people can cope without these drugs; why can't you? The drugs cause an overall flattening of mood, which leaves you not as distressed but also not able to feel very much of anything. Then there are the side-effects, ranging from the inconvenient to the horrific. Claims by drug companies that newer, more expensive drugs have fewer side-effects and are more effective are not convincing in the light of previous claims for older 'wonder' drugs that are now acknowledged to be harmful.

There are other ways of relieving sadness than prescription drugs: physical exercise, being with friends, meditation, pets – whatever gets you through it (which will be different for everyone). By medicalising it, the possibilities are drastically narrowed.

There is a wider issue here: there seems to be an expectation within our society that happiness is the ultimate goal. There is also an expectation, fuelled by the dominant scientific-world view, that there is a solution for every problem (and the mental *illness* model clearly implies that there is a 'cure', which is what people with a mental illness label are expected to want). It seems to me that these two attitudes lie behind the dominance of the medical mental illness model – the search for 'quick-fix' solutions to unhappiness.

Colin tells us that he hides his real feelings from friends and people he knows, because if he really lets them know how badly he is feeling they would just tell him to pull himself together. Feeling terrible is not 'normal'; you're not supposed to display despair to other people. Everyone wants to be happy. The solution is to see unhappiness as an illness: we can then hand over responsibility for dealing with people with depression to specially-trained 'experts': the mental health professionals.

It is often a relief for people with depression to hand over responsibility for their needs to the professionals. Sometimes you need to give up control over your own life for a time. But the mental illness model does not promote the idea of the individual taking back control once ready to do so. Although it promotes the *idea* of a cure, in reality it promotes permanent dependency. It keeps responsibility firmly in the hands of mental health professionals.

Many mental health service users who accept the mental illness model find it threatening for this model to be challenged. Indeed, Colin uses the concept to validate his own feelings of vulnerability. If you have a mental illness, people have to take your problems seriously. If the concept of mental illness is ditched, then what are you left with? There is the fear that you will be blamed for not coping with your problems, or, worse, there will be the presumption that there was never a real problem in the first place – in which case you're just a malingerer.

The Bradford Home Treatment Service, where I work, acknowledges the fact that many service users experience psychiatry as oppressive, and strives to create a more equal relationship between mental health professionals and service users. A key factor in trying to achieve this is that we do not use diagnostic categories; we focus instead on people's needs as individuals, trying to provide the support they feel will be most helpful. This may involve practical help with benefits and housing, support with improving social networks or simply giving people a chance to talk. It may include short-term use of medication too. The emphasis is on handing back responsibility to the service user as soon as (but not until) the person feels ready to take it. Service users feel this non-medical approach is much more helpful than traditional psychiatry. The service has been awarded 'Beacon' status as an example of best practice within the NHS. The point is that this service can provide the help and support people need without dismissing the seriousness of their difficulties and without using the mental illness model. So why use the concept at all?

Like Kate Millett, who wrote *The Loony-bin Trip*, and like Colin, I was given a diagnosis of depression. I know what it feels like to lock yourself away from the world, barricading yourself within the safe-seeming womb of your room. I was absorbed into the mental health system, unemployed and considered unemployable, for over 15 years, until I eventually found a job where it was a requirement, instead of a liability, to be a user of mental health services. It is only since joining the Bradford Home Treatment Team as service user development worker that I came across accounts such as Kate Millett's, which challenge traditional, medical psychiatry.

For me personally, the discovery that there are alternatives to the mental illness model, alternative ways of framing my own experience of distress, came as a revelation. Nevertheless, the defining of deep-seated unhappiness as an illness is something that, on a personal level, I still find myself continually struggling with. I need to retreat into a place of helplessness sometimes, and the idea of being 'ill' bolsters that.

I hope that this commentary is seen by the writer of the account as helpful. Even though my perspective is different from his, we have in common similar experiences of distress. In the end, what really matters is that mental health service users get the help and support we need to move on with our lives, rather than being given what mental health professionals think we need.

'The question is not how to get cured, but how to live.' Joseph Conrad (1900)

Resistance is useless

Lizzie Gardiner

I haven't had a day as low as this for a while. I don't want to do anything but neither can I bear to be still. I've only minimal concentration and I can't find a spot to stand comfortably in my own boots. I'm beyond consolation, I'm unresponsive and I can't follow the track of a conversation. I find it impossible to come up with all the usual platitudes for kind and enquiring folk and I haven't answered the phone all day. I feel unwell, without any symptoms of physical illness, but with all the gloom and discomfort of a polar bear in a sauna.

There are lots of things that I would have liked to have done today, but I have about as much chance of lobotomising the Pope as I do of starting, let alone finishing them. This is a day when all I can do is wait. I got the children to school because I always do. But I came home again to immediately find that all my responses to the world felt just too big and intense. I took to my bed and slept most of the day.

On days like today I endure the continual feeling that I should be somewhere else, doing something I've forgotten to do or not doing the things that I am. I feel as though I exist in a universe that only sometimes collides with the one everybody else inhabits. Death is just behind me, waiting as always for a lapse in concentration or a poor footing.

Previous experience has established that although the vultures do circle on a day like today, they rarely land. I have learnt that this blip doesn't mean much in the big picture and that it has little connection to any particular worry or issue. I know that evasive action can, but may well not, work and that it's pointless to analyse or talk. There is nothing in the world that will make me feel any better until I just do. Resistance is indeed useless but I don't have to be a passive victim of my illness.

I use writing as an important part of managing my symptoms. It's the most powerful way I have to externalise my experience and the repetitive action of typing is useful for occupying the more easily led parts of my brain. I kept everything inside before I became depressed and it really didn't work. Writing gives me a focus now and a tangible anchor for my turbulent thoughts and feelings. It's often the only way I can afford to be completely honest.

I continue to write when I'm low, as must be apparent. On a day like this I pour out whatever comes to mind and then come back to decipher it when I'm better able to govern my thoughts. I might only spend ten minutes at the computer, depending on my concentration and the mercy of the children. I might sit down to write several times a day. I've learned to accept that I'm easily distracted and that there's still no law requiring an intelligible first draft.

I spend a lot of my time fending off the spectral bullies of 'uselessness' and 'hopelessness'. Writing gives me a barricade behind which to hide – in that I've produced something. During work on this piece I've had to cajole and bribe myself into working, because although procrastination will find any number of things to take greater priority, I do know that the satisfaction and pleasure of having written something is of great benefit to me.

Writing serves all sorts of purposes. It's a safe place to leave my internal life when it gets too scary to carry about with me. It's a comfortable way to communicate with the outside world if I can't bear to do it in person. It's something that I've grown able to feel good at and it's something I can do to help myself.

There's nothing like a serious bout of depression to make you take stock. I've had to re-evaluate, re-think and re-design my life right down to the basics. I've had to find ways to monitor and manage my symptoms. It's been my good fortune to be treated by a psychologist who had the perception to realise that my natural inclination to write might prove a powerful weapon for me and he spent months gaining my confidence to the point when I'd show him my work. He's since encouraged and practically helped me to become increasingly able to make some sense of my depression through my writing and to regain an overall sense of purpose, contribution and equilibrium. Now I can tolerate a day like today.

POEMS

V. I. Oliver

Song

Daddy was a bugger, he was buggered as a boy
Took the hatred out on me, used me as a toy
But I can take, take it, take it
Spread around some joy
Daddy, Daddy, you bastard, you're dead.

Daddy died alone and guilty, took his secret to the grave
Turned to Jesus at the last, tried to get himself saved
Didn't know I had it in me to be this bloody brave
Daddy, Daddy, you bastard, you're dead.

Now Daddy was the first one to teach me loving touch
There was joy and laughter too, but that buggery hurt so much
I've used people all my life as a prop and as a crutch
Trying to give something back.

Now to live in my body, I have to love my Dad
'Cos his was the first loving touch that I ever had
That language isn't mine – that is what really made me mad
I need words like air.

Daddy smelt when he was dying, smelled that smell for years and years
Someday I may let it go, and really cry the tears
But the love there is between us helped me drive away the fear
Oh, my dear.

So if you've been hated, if someone's shat on you
Look for the grain of love in them, it just might see you through
'Cos each of us is sacred – that means you, and you, and you
And – maybe my Daddy, too.

Untitled

The audience waits, medical students about to (they hope) see a
soul dissected in the way they themselves once dissected rats.

I enter. I am aware of the Professor, of them, of their interest and
Their boredom. A simmering rage at the humiliation, scorn at their presuming to
Understand, rage at my impotence – all comes out as
Gibberish. It is clear that wherever my reality lies, it is not here. But this
Is happening to me.

Questions: a sense of someone reaching out to my inner space to
Meet me. But to meet me not in order to rescue me, but to tag, label,
Identify. I am a process, an item in a taxonomy, not someone to meet.
This, not the humiliation, was the real betrayal.

Untitled

Our women, myself included,
Have been approached, while psychiatric patients,
By males of similar status
And asked to become prostitutes.
I'm speculating.
But it seems plausible that
Feeling keenly the shame of their position,
These men sought to re-establish themselves,
To raise their self-esteem,
In the most commonplace, most "normal", most so called normal,
Most degrading way possible:–
By making a woman a slave.

Wrapper

The floor is covered in squares. Each square has a meaning. The
Whole floor speaks of division and divisiveness.
How to understand this space, this floor on which I crawl,
Dribbling from the drugs?
The chewing-gum wrapper says "Please dispose of this wrapper thoughtfully".
That word. Thoughtful. I have always been thoughtful. I have
Always been thoughtful in the social sense, how to be thoughtful about my situation now, this floor, this wrapper.
This space is dangerous: doctors are supposed to be helping me.
Why does my vision now only contain a floor and a wrapper.
Why are they both so important?
Meaning, significance, symbols. In this space. In this here and
Now, no-one can reach me. It seemed. It seemed I had a choice, that between this and death by suicide.
This has meaning.
It is meaning I need.
So, if there is no meaning, I invent one.
I am resourceful.
This knowledge is necessary.

Gratitude (for a Ward Sister)

I kicked her shin.
Hard.
It was intended to hurt, and it did.
I watched the anger and the pain in her face.
Waited.
Watched her reach instead for her much-in-demand compassion,
Saw her put who and where I was, first,
As she reached out her arms and said
"I think you need a hug".

Fiona Shaw, in her book *Out of Me* (1997), the story of a postnatal breakdown, comments on the process of writing about her own mental illness. She wrote:

> 'When I began writing this book, I did so in the effort to shore myself up against the whirling chaos of my mind. I was in fear of disintegration, though I couldn't, and still can't describe what I mean by that. I had no idea that my terror would give birth to a book. What has been important has been the act of turning blankness and confusion into narrative coherence.'

Fiona Shaw's statement, I think, captures one of the fundamental reasons for writing out of a personal experience of mental illness. The aim seems to be to gain internal coherence from the structure that a narrative account bestows on what, especially in the psychoses, must undoubtedly be a terrifying and disturbing experience. Her account is in the tradition of Daniel Schreber's *Memoirs of my Nervous Illness* (1955), William Styron's *Darkness Visible* (1991), Tim Lott's *The Scent of Dried Roses* (1996) and Lewis Wolpert's *Malignant Sadness* (1999).

These writers all approach their experiences, using the autobiographical method, to examine the nature of mental phenomena and the origins (both moral and instrumental) of mental illness, and attempt to locate and name the meaning of these experiences. In essence, the authors try to make sense of a disruptive personal experience. These accounts succeed partly because the orderly structure and the reasonableness of the arguments reassure us that the authors have not succumbed to the virulent experiences. However, Sarah Ferguson's *A Guard Within* (1973), an autobiographical account that is a concentrated outpouring of misery and hopelessness, which is deeply insightful and masterly in its control of language but ultimately overpowering in its despair and anguish, succeeds for other reasons. It succeeds, I believe, because it satisfies our curiosity of what the depths of melancholia can be like.

The straight autobiographical genre is only one of many possible ways of writing about one's experience of different mental phenomena. Other narrative modes, for example the autobiographical novel, such as Janet Frame's *Faces in the Water* (1961) and Sylvia Plath's *The Bell Jar* (1963), allow the authors greater freedom in exploring their experiences. The literary material derived from memory is bent and sculpted by imagination in the service of a plot, a story line. In ascribing the various experiences to fictitious characters, the writer gains a degree of detachment from the personal experience. As one would say in psychiatry, the personal and subjective become objectified. There is the risk that the deviant and terrifying will be rendered mythical and elevated to a romanticised account.

Janet Frame, in her autobiographical novel, wrote:

'There is an aspect of madness which is seldomed mentioned in fiction because it would damage the romantic popular idea of the insane as a person whose speech appears as immediately poetic.'

Thus, for Frame the totality of what it is to be mentally ill must be the subject of literary treatment. Those situations in which the subject's behaviour affronted or caused uneasiness, when the subjects wept or moaned, quarrelled or complained, must all be represented in literature. Frame's intention is to use an autobiographical but fictional structure to ensure that her account retains a literary integrity, that is, that it is faithful to the reality that she is trying to describe.

If she had written a plain autobiography, I believe that it would have been more difficult for her to describe her own situation in a way that retains that admirable capacity for harsh honesty without doing untold damage to her own self-esteem. Also, the autobiographical novel retains the smell and texture of real life but is tempered by the fact that the all too painful emotions serve the purpose of a story, which is over and above the experiences themselves. Thus, these experiences act as they do in real life, they occur within the fabric of a life. What literature does is to allow the possibility for others to share vicariously in the life of the literary characters, and perhaps to start to empathise with their dilemma. Literature, when it is successful, reduces the emotional distance between the protagonists and us, and in doing this opens the way for imagining the life of the other.

Poetry is an entirely different dimension as the vehicle for exploring personal experience of mental illness. By definition it is as much about the form of language as it is about the content. Meaning is derived from rhythm, melody, prosody and the subtle deployment of the ambiguities inherent in language, and modern European poetry's particular preoccupation with the intensely personal makes poetry an attractive medium for the communication of personal emotional distress.

Both Lizzie's and V. I. Oliver's contributions confront writing about the inner turmoil, the disturbances of thinking and perception, but perhaps more importantly the experience of being subject to the scrutiny of others. These poems, with economy and directness and an unwavering gaze, confront us with disquieting and troubling situations, and draw us in such that we cannot ignore what is the other's pervasive humanity. And that is the strength of all literature. By the subtle arrangement of words, we come to be charged with the appropriate emotions such that the humanity of the other's situation becomes patent. The mistreatment of individuals suffering from mental illness becomes possible only when their humanity is not transparently obvious.

Mental illness and employment

Kay McKall

I remember I argued with the psychiatrist, unwilling to accept such an unwelcome diagnosis. I had always viewed myself as a strong personality, and strong personalities didn't succumb to depression. That only affected ineffectual non-copers; surely that couldn't be me.

It had started so innocuously ten months before, with waking at four every morning. It was annoying but nothing more. Of course I knew that waking so early was associated with depression, but I wasn't depressed – I was busy and involved both socially and as a full-time GP.

But somehow the job seemed to get harder. The patients seemed more demanding. They irritated me. I tried to jolly myself along; if that cantankerous old dear in the next village insisted on a visit, I'd drop into the garden centre on the way back. More than five extra patients to see at the end of surgery earned a chocolate bar.

Chocolate bars, however, couldn't stop this growing wave of negativity. I felt increasingly overwhelmed by patients and their seemingly unreasonable demands. Each time I saw an extra, before saying a word to the patient, I reached for a red pen, wrote 'Emergency' on the notes and slowly and deliberately drew a red box around it. Anything short of crushing central chest pain I considered trivial and time-wasting. I received the first complaint of my career – for rudeness.

I woke at three every morning.

My chief aim in medical practice became getting the patient out of the chair and out of the door. Several times, appalled by my own sloppiness, I phoned patients and asked them to return for proper examinations rather than a bum's rush. But only every now and again. The effort seemed too great and what was the point anyway?

I hated myself like this. I kept telling myself to settle down and assume at least an outward face of equanimity. I consciously acted the part of a caring interested doctor, but all too frequently the bile would erupt through.

Negativity contaminated my personal life. Away from work I was demanding and unreasonable. I offended and annoyed friends.

I woke at two every morning.

I felt as if I was in an airplane whose controls weren't working. I kept sinking towards the ground, sometimes by enormous effort regaining control and gaining some height, but soon drifting inexorably down again. I could see the ground approaching ever more rapidly as what remained of my personality disintegrated. I could no longer meet the gaze of patients without my own eyes filling with tears.

I renounced my closest and dearest friends. I was beyond their reach and they were beyond mine. I was too agitated to sleep.

During the final spiral dive into the ground I hardly knew what was happening. The world had receded from me. I was a wraith-like alien in a world filled with normal people. Nothing mattered; food, appearance, money, reputation, image were all of no importance. I was hollow, devoid of thoughts or character. I felt I must be invisible.

I drove into work one Monday morning, looked at the appointment book and the visit list, and walked out.

At home I stood staring out into the back garden, dank and lifeless with late winter. I had come to the end of my natural life. The thought didn't upset me. I had left emotions behind. I couldn't see any way forward, nor did I see any point in trying.

But the phone and the doorbell kept ringing. People seemed to be so upset. I couldn't see why. In a way it made me feel worse. I had caused these nice normal people to become unhappy; another weight of guilt was added to my load. I had to make some kind of effort. As I dialled the number of our sector psychiatrist, my doctor persona emerged and I informed him breezily that I was having a little trouble, don't we all, those patients drive you crazy ha ha. He agreed to see me the next day.

Going to see him made me feel even more inadequate. What a fuss I was making over nothing; what a useless neurotic I was.

I told him my problem was just failure to cope with work stress. He suggested crisply that I stick to my symptoms and leave the diagnosis to him.

The load that was lifted with that – that of being a sensible doctor and 'one of the guys' – was unimaginable. I sat hunched on the edge of his sofa, sobbing and shaking and wringing my hands as I tried to tell my story.

The psychiatrist was amazed. I was so obviously depressed.

It was a bombshell to me. It had never once occurred to me that I might have a psychiatric illness. And what an illness. It reeked of limp-wristedness and an inability to cope with life. Sad people who sucked a little vitality out of each person they came into contact with.

Then it dawned on me that he was offering both a diagnosis and a cure. It all seemed too easy, too miraculous. Could all the misery be reversed with a pill? I felt as if I'd hit the ground in my airplane but the ground had turned into a cloud and I was safely out of the other side.

Since then there have been some swooping ups and downs, caused chiefly by ineffective drugs, non-compliance and my amazing lack of insight. The episodes of jollity I had always taken for granted have now been labelled hypomania. I visited my psychiatrist while in this wildly expansive mood and rather startled him. It also slowly became clear to me that I'd been struggling under the weight of this illness most of my life.

Now I take lithium and an antidepressant and I look forward to the next day for the time first I can remember. Is this normal? Is this how other people feel all the time? I honestly don't know, having spent my life inside my manic-depressive brain. But if they do, they have no idea how lucky they are.

COMMENTARY – ALISON COBB

Employment discrimination is a common experience for people with a mental illness diagnosis and it is important to remember that people do resume working in demanding, responsible jobs in which their colleagues and clients are glad to see them back. It is worth, however, looking at the extent of exclusion and what can be done to counter it.

Exclusion from employment

Once it is known that someone has had psychiatric treatment he or she may find his or her whole credibility as a person undermined or be treated with apprehension.

'When I had to tell [my boss] I was being taken into hospital his reaction said it all. He sat back in his seat wanting to keep as far away from me as possible. As soon as mental illness is mentioned people literally back off from you.' (Dunn & Crawford, 1999)

Only eighteen per cent of people diagnosed with a mental illness have jobs (estimates from the Labour Force Survey, 2000 (see http://www.statistics.gov.uk/http://www.statistics.gov.uk/)). When Mind invited people in its networks to report experiences of discrimination, abuse or harassment the largest problem they identified was employment. Thirty-eight per cent of the 778 respondents had been harassed, intimidated or teased at work and thirty-four per cent were forced to resign or were dismissed. One in five of these people had been employed as a nurse or in another caring profession, or had been an NHS employee. Fifty-two per cent said they had had to conceal their psychiatric history for fear of losing their job. Sixty-nine per cent had been put off applying for jobs for fear of unfair treatment.

Such rejection is especially hard when a person has already had his or her confidence and sense of self-worth damaged, or when he/she has come through the experience stronger and more empathic.

Telling the employer (or not)

The decision about what to say to whom about your experience of mental distress is of course very personal. Once said, there is no unsaying it. Here is a summary of the potential risks and benefits of disclosure to think about when developing a strategy on how to handle it (Extract from *Mind Guide to Surviving Working Life*; Cobb, 2000).

The potential risks of disclosing something about your mental health history include:

- not getting the job
- teasing or harassment from other employees
- being assumed to be a less productive member of the team
- fewer opportunities for career development
- being treated as more vulnerable than other employees or having everything – anger, excitement, an 'off day', time off sick, a grievance – put down to mental illness
- coming under closer scrutiny than other employees and having to work harder to gain the same respect.

Potential benefits of disclosure are:

- being 'out' at work can encourage others in the same situation
- keeping it secret may be too stressful, or against your beliefs
- it gives you a basis for requesting adjustments to your job or work environment
- it could open the way for involving an outside adviser or support worker who could see you at work or speak directly with your employer
- it could make it easier to go into work at times when your symptoms are greater
- it enables you to enlist the support of colleagues.

Employers' responsibilities

Employees and applicants have to make their own decisions about disclosure, but what an employer can do is create a work environment where it is safe to be open about mental ill health. This means making it clear that equal opportunity and disability policies include people with mental health problems. As employers' guidance states:

> 'If it is known that there is a willingness to make reasonable adjustments for all disabled applicants and employees, people with mental health problems will be much more likely to trust the employer and colleagues and be open. Acceptance is morale-boosting; fear of being 'found out' can be stressful and sap confidence.' (Employers' Forum on Disability, 1998)

The employment duties under the Disability Discrimination Act 1995 are not to treat applicants and employees with disabilities less favourably than others, and to make reasonable adjustments if an applicant or employee with a disability is at a substantial disadvantage in relation to others. Learning not to make assumptions about people on the basis of a mental illness diagnosis is at the heart of anti-discriminatory practice.

The Disability Discrimination Act case of Watkiss v John Laing plc (2000) shows how blanket assumptions can result in discrimination. The most qualified candidate for a senior post was offered the job subject to a medical examination but had the offer withdrawn on medical grounds when he disclosed a diagnosis of schizophrenia, despite saying that he had successfully managed his mental health for eight years. The company did not seek further medical advice and did not discuss it with the candidate or his current employer. The rejection was based on the candidate's mental health history and not his ability to do the job.

An employee with mental health problems may, but will not necessarily, need adjustments to be made. Examples include:

- a gradual return to work after time off sick
- quiet workspace or working from home
- adjustments to hours, for example, to accommodate medical appointments or medication effects
- supportive supervision.

What information and support do employers need?

Although the media's association of mental illness with violence is very pervasive, employers' worries are most likely to be about the person's capacity to do the job. One research study found that a person with depression had significantly reduced chances of employment compared to someone with diabetes because of concerns about poor work performance (Glozier, 1998).

It is important, therefore, that employers have ready access to information on the realities of mental distress to allay unwarranted fears. They also need support and information about what work adjustments might be needed by a person with mental health problems, and what to do when they are worried about an employee's mental health. There is no reason to expect employers to be experts in mental illness; what matters is that they know where they can get assistance when they need it.

The role of mental health professionals and agencies

There are several ways in which mental health professionals and agencies can contribute to people's prospects of successful employment.
As employers:

- recognise the value of experience of mental distress to mental health work
- take a lead in best employment practices.

As providers:

- develop employment support services and other schemes to increase work opportunities for people with mental health problems
- work with individuals in recognising and responding to their work aspirations
- respond to employers' needs for information, advice and support.

In this way mental health professionals can help people in mental distress gain or retain a sense of a future that involves working, and also help give employers the confidence to employ people who experience mental distress.

Stephen Dominic

When I was first diagnosed with schizophrenia twelve years ago, I was extremely angry. The diagnosis made any hope of a progressive recovery seem even less likely. Today, if someone asks me what schizophrenia means, I cannot begin to explain. I say 'my diagnosis is schizophrenia', with the implicit meaning that 'it is somebody else who has diagnosed me as this', but I would not say 'I am a schizophrenic'. In other words, I still have not completely accepted the diagnosis or the word. However, it haunts me every day. The word schizophrenia is so much a part of my psyche that I almost feel as if I belong to a schizophrenic family of people in society who are diagnosed the same way as I am.

In spite of this I no longer feel 'outside' schizophrenia but 'inside' it. There are many people who are 'outside' schizophrenia and they are easy to recognise and to notice. People 'outside' schizophrenia possess, express and react to schizophrenia in a recognisable way; they have an in-built fear, ignorant rejection, a formula that suggests a schizophrenic is a 'madman', a 'split personality', a danger to society. This is only a selection of people's views towards the condition. This is the reason why I was angry when I was first diagnosed with schizophrenia because when I was diagnosed, my intellectual experience of the disease was still 'outside' schizophrenia, although my mental and physical behaviour suggested I was 'inside' it.

I use these terms because suffering from the disease is like being a prisoner in oneself, unable to explain how you genuinely feel, how you genuinely think, constantly detached from the world that once upon a time you used to inhabit.

I am on the inside and the rest of the world is on the outside. I am still trying to break out but, in the case of a person diagnosed with schizophrenia, there is no fixed term for release, no remission, no Home Secretary to give you a judicial review, no one with the keys to open the door to a life you once had.

I am still haunted by images, people and words of an intense period of my life that happened over eighteen years ago. These images appear to me every day, although I am able to deal with them better now than I did before.

However, I still feel detached from people to the extent that 'I do not speak their language'. I feel fraudulent, as if I am living a lie, and in a twilight zone of fact and fiction where I cannot properly distinguish the two. This state of mind is something that has been forced upon me. In front of the judge I would say 'Yes, I am completely innocent of the charges but at the same time I am completely guilty. And I ask the judge for his understanding.'

It is the frustration of not being able to properly come to terms with one's own experiences. Not being able to properly rationalise. This is being inside schizophrenia and in this respect I have become more aware of how schizophrenia is treated by those on the outside. I feel as if I am part of a discriminated minority, rejected by all those on the outside. People, however, are fed information and they believe that information, and I have extremely strong views about how schizophrenia is treated in the media.

This year three thousand people will die on our roads. Not one of those deaths will be registered in blazing headlines on the front page of a national newspaper. However, if one person with schizophrenia kills someone as a result of their illness, depending on the importance of the case, it will get front-page treatment or national news coverage on television. All the language used, the views and presentation of the reports made about a person suffering from schizophrenia or another mental illness is in the style of those on the outside.

Even papers such as the *Mirror*, which has no hesitation in defending the National Health Service (NHS), would have no hesitation in using headlines such as 'schizo butchers' and in expressive language detail what the 'schizo' did. It is my argument that such papers care more for the NHS than for those people who use it. People with schizophrenia are patients in the NHS.

Another example of media denigration of people with mental health problems was the case of Michael Stone. The judicial opinion of some of the tabloid papers was that anyone suffering from mental illness, who is regarded as a danger to society, should be incarcerated on a permanent basis until such time as he or she is seen as 'safe' to be released. In our system of justice, even people who have been imprisoned for committing murder can be released after fourteen years. Why, because you happen to suffer from mental illness, is it suggested you must be permanently imprisoned even when you have not committed a crime? That is the justice of the barbarian.

The same people believe it is wrong to take a tough line on speeding offences: do people suffering from a mental illness kill three thousand people a year? But the media and politicians are not concerned with people's lives, because life is cheap. They care more for the way in which people die. A man killed on the road is not news, although it's a life. A man killed by a person with schizophrenia is news, because it sells copy. The media and politicians have no sense of how much damage they do in their senseless reporting and their twisted logic, the logic of the people on the outside. They have no idea of how they diminish the chances of recovery of those suffering from mental illness, and no idea of how they prevent them from restoring their lives. No idea of how they hinder the thousands of people in support services who fight these debilitating diseases on a daily basis.

I know what I am talking about because I am talking from the inside.

COMMENTARY – PETER BYRNE

Stephen is angry that the word schizophrenia does not begin to describe his experiences over the past eighteen years. For him, the word is a life sentence, and removes any hope of recovery. Despite this, he is 'locked' inside schizophrenia, away from the world outside. This separation of them, 'the schizophrenics', from us, 'non-schizophrenics', is a creation of society. The formula states that someone with this condition is a madman, is dangerous, or has a split personality. The language of the newspapers is 'in the style of those on the outside', loaded with danger and threat, making headlines with stories that meet the requirements of the formula. The newspapers themselves are inconsistent. The *Mirror* supports the NHS, but ignores the difficulties of the 'schizos' who use this service. The *Daily Mail* calls for the indefinite incarceration of dangerous mentally ill people, but ignores the three thousand dead on the roads when it campaigns for a softer line on speeding offences. It isn't just the inconsistency of these two newspapers – it is that they use scare tactics to keep people like Stephen locked in a state of schizophrenia.

There have always been problems with the word schizophrenia. At almost every user meeting I have attended, someone – usually a relative fed up with the adverse publicity – suggests we change it. It was devised to describe the splitting of the functions of the brain: how we experience perceptions or how we develop an idea. The trouble is, it is often wrongly described as a split personality. What the public believes to be schizophrenia owes more to Stephenson's Jekyll and Hyde (published in 1886) than to a century of scientific research. Jekyll and Hyde stories sell newspapers. Tales of men out of control, normal one minute but violently insane the next, excite the public's imagination. If someone commits a crime we do not understand, he or she must be hiding an insane darker side. For sane/insane we read normal/violent. The madmen may look like us, but under all that normal stuff, they're crazy, ready to pounce. This is the real media formula. Understanding mental illness is hard work. Demonising the people who have it is easy. The logic of the media is to play to a prejudice that has been around for centuries. The public likes to feel protected from people who used to be locked away in asylums. Besides which, they don't answer back.

But the real issue here isn't a psychiatrist writing another 'the media is to blame' piece. Schizophrenia affects up to one per cent of the population, men and women of any culture, every class and regardless of age. But society's response makes people like Stephen feel like a criminal. He is bombarded with negative images of this illness, and instead of being encouraged to seek support, he feels 'fraudulent', unable to speak the language of people who do not have this condition. In many ways he is trapped in the discourse that mental illness is untreatable and uncontrollable. His crime is to have schizophrenia. At a time when he needs the support of people around him to help him understand what is happening, the word/formula/logic of schizophrenia cuts him off from that support. He is thrown into a discriminated minority, rejected by those on the outside. That's the part no one can explain.

PERSONAL STORIES

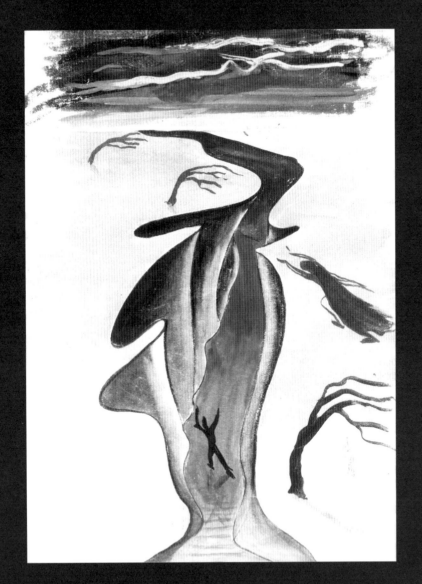

From the Adamson Collection

Mental illness affects people in different ways. It can creep up insidiously in the form of deepening depression, undiagnosed and untreated, enveloping the individual in a fog of despair and feelings of worthlessness.

Conversely it can appear seemingly out of the blue as happened in my case when puerperal psychosis struck after the birth of a much wanted second child when I was twenty-eight years old.

I was full of energy and joy for the first five days after the birth. With hindsight I would say that I was euphoric, or hypomanic, but at the time this condition was not recognised by the professionals involved in prenatal and postnatal care. I had been extremely fit all through the pregnancy and worked three mornings a week as a remedial reading teacher, as well as representing junior teachers throughout Wales for my professional union, the National Union of Teachers (NUT). This involved regular committee meetings in London and chairing a conference of young teachers in Wales when six months pregnant. I appeared to be in a stable marriage, had a gorgeous toddler of 21 months, excellent childcare and the option to continue to teach part-time while developing a long-term interest in equal opportunities within the NUT.

So what went wrong and why did it happen to me? I asked this question many times over as this nameless illness took over my whole existence, wrecking relationships and friendships, almost robbing me of my children and home, and leaving me with a job at a time of full employment, but without a career.

On the sixth day after the birth I had to go to the supermarket to stock up the cupboard supplies, which had run down in the time that I had been in hospital. I set off for the nearest town aware that something was wrong and that I was feeling distant from all that was happening around me. I put this down to the tiredness that one feels after childbirth, as I had no close family support. Also, there was a requirement to resume the normal role of a married woman in the mid-1960s; we were expected to run a home and rear children without any lowering of standards, while at the same time get the satisfaction from either full- or part-time work where one knew one's skills and training would be used. Perhaps I wanted too much too quickly.

In the supermarket things went from bad to worse and I was aware of taking things from the shelves without knowing what they were or what I needed. I managed to struggle back to the car, drove home and was put to bed. I ceased to eat or drink and stopped talking to anyone. All seemed hopeless and pointless and I didn't want to live.

I was admitted to the local psychiatric hospital under the Mental Health Act and treated with a variety of drugs. No one gave me a diagnosis, no one gave me any information about how to manage the medication effectively and as I was on a Section, no one told me when I would be able to go home and be reunited with my children again – or if I would ever go home again. Finally I was persuaded by my then husband to accept electroconvulsive therapy (ECT) if I wanted to be released from the Section. Being in a position where effectively any free choice was not available, I reluctantly signed for the treatment. ECT gave me a headache, affected my memory and did little to alleviate my depression, but it did mean that I was released from the Section and allowed to leave hospital so that I could be reunited with my two children after six months in hospital.

As I continued to have episode after episode of this mystery illness that had no diagnosis, my confidence was shattered and at one point I was suicidal. To be told to 'pull yourself together' or 'think what you are doing to your family' pushed me further into depression. Some friends disappeared, my marriage ended and my career as a teacher was jeopardised. Bizarre behaviour during the manic phases of the illness was almost impossible to explain once I was stable again and apologies were seldom accepted.

The turning point came with a change of psychiatrist after I had rejected the system of meaningless three-monthly appointments with the repeated series of questions asked by the original consultant. This had in no way given me the answers that I needed or the diagnosis that should have been my right. The system also appeared paternalistic. I was not allowed to ask questions, handle my own medication in an informed way or move towards the smallest form of self-management. I opted out of the system and became a 'non-complier'. It seemed to work for me for a time but, with hindsight, as a working single parent I was 'up in an airplane without a parachute'.

A summons from the new psychiatrist who took over my care and was irritated by the cavalier way in which I ignored appointments brought me to heel. Via his secretary he warned me that if I ignored the next appointment he would cross me off his list. Then, when I needed his help, and as he said 'I would surely need his help again', he would not be available.

Mutinous at this ultimatum, I nevertheless grudgingly kept the appointment and from that first unpromising meeting my life was turned round. I was given the correct diagnosis of manic depression, not schizophrenia, and put on the appropriate medication, lithium. The diagnosis (not label) gave me back normality and ensured that I tailored my lifestyle in such a way as to avoid stressful situations and people. I took regular exercise and ate and drank sensibly. To my wail of 'can't I even drink red wine?' came the reply, 'just be sensible'. No paternalism there.

My two children gave me tremendous support, handling my occasional attacks of mania with great maturity all through their adolescence. My son dealt with psychiatrists and hospital admissions without the help of a twenty-four-hour crisis line or appointed keyworker. When he went to university, my daughter coped with one attack while taking her A-level exams. Both my children had a healthy semi-detached attitude to my manic depressive bouts, dealing with any problem as it arose but getting on with their lives in the knowledge that I had a superb professional working with me towards my managing the illness effectively, as I ultimately learnt to do. They never looked on themselves as 'carers', they just cared enough to let me manage the illness effectively on my own.

The psychiatrist who turned the illness around for me was consistently overworked but still prepared to give an hour or more of his time to patients at crucial stages of their illness when the need to talk was paramount and would not fit into a ten minute slot every three months. An impending crisis would be dealt with, initially in my case, by a short voluntary admission and later by self-medication and a few days off from school. Time spent talking to me and identifying trigger factors paid off in the long-term as I no longer needed expensive hospital treatment or regular out-patient appointments. Diagnosis, self-management and a balanced partnership forged from mutual respect returned me to a normal life.

After thirty years as a primary school teacher I am now a part-time lecturer in mental illness to professionals, have worked as a lay assessor for the Social Services Inspectorate at the Welsh Office and set up the Manic Depression Wales Office. You could call me the ultimate late developer.

Most importantly I have a full and enjoyable life secure in the knowledge that I am able to manage this major psychotic illness effectively on my own. As Bob Hoskins said in the BT advertisement, 'It's good to talk.' In my case talking to the right professional at the right time was a life saver.

COMMENTARY – MILES RINALDI

Manic depression is a serious mental health problem involving extreme swings of mood (highs and lows). Manic depression is also known as bipolar affective disorder. Both men and women of any age from adolescence onwards and from any social or ethnic background can develop manic depression. One in a hundred people will be affected by manic depression at some time in their life.

It often first occurs when work, study, family or emotional pressures are at their greatest. In women it can also be triggered by childbirth or during the menopause.

The illness is episodic (occurs in phases). It is possible to remain well for long periods of time. Typically the key to coping with manic depression is an early diagnosis and acceptance of the condition. From this point, a person can take up self-management, health care, therapy and medication as appropriate. Medication is frequently prescribed, most commonly a mood stabiliser such as lithium. Talking treatments such as cognitive–behavioural therapy (CBT) can also be useful, although this may be difficult to access through the NHS. Severe or untreated episodes of manic depression can be very damaging for individuals and their friends and families.

Although much progress has been made in understanding manic depression and how to manage it, research has not led to a consensus on either the cause or cure. Some research suggests that there is, if not a known genetic link, then certainly an inherited predisposition to developing manic depression. We also know that stressful life events often precede an episode of mania or depression.

Self-management

Self-management is one way of coping with manic depression; it is not the answer, but it can play a powerful role in the management of the illness. Research has shown that self-management is an invaluable part of stabilising the condition. The self-management training programme is built on the following principle: 'People with manic depression can become the experts on their own mental health.' A key resource is the personal experience and knowledge that each person brings to the course.

The Manic Depression Fellowship's self-management training programme was written by people who themselves have a diagnosis of manic depression, and is continuously improved and up-dated to reflect feedback and information from the course participants about their particular experiences. The facilitators who deliver the programme also have a diagnosis of manic depression, and have learned to use self-management effectively.

The self-management training programme is user led and run. The programme aims to help participants to develop new strategies, monitor their mood states, link thoughts, feelings and behaviours, and to become alert to mood variations. Facilitators act as role models for participants, demonstrating and sharing the personal experiences and knowledge that have allowed them to gain confidence in taking control of their own lives. Self-management involves learning to recognise early triggers and warning signs of an episode and devising an action plan to prevent or minimise severe mood swings. Perry and co-workers (1999) found that improved social function and performance in employment resulted if people were taught to recognise the trigger to their illness and to seek early treatment.

The Manic Depression Fellowship's self-management training programme is based on the following assumptions:

- hope: people with manic depression are not 'ill' all of the time. They stay 'well' for long periods of time and are able to do what they want with their lives
- personal responsibility: self-management is the process of taking control of one's life through acknowledging personal responsibility. Users can become active agents in managing their lives rather than passive recipients of treatment
- self-advocacy: this is having belief in oneself, knowing one's rights, getting the facts, planning a strategy, gathering support, targeting one's efforts, expressing oneself clearly and being assertive. The self-management training programme is built on the following principle: people with manic depression can become the experts on their own mental health
- education: the need for knowledge is broad, for example, from informing oneself about medication, to looking at lifestyle, careers and leisure activities.

The course is delivered over six weekly sessions of two-and-a-half hours each or a residential weekend, incorporating a mixture of presentations, discussions and participatory exercises.

The Manic Depression Fellowship chooses to use two images to illustrate the connections between the components of a self-management training programme. The image of a jigsaw is used to show that self-management consists of many techniques. Each person may decide not only how many pieces there are but also which are the appropriate ones to use.

The other image is a set of traffic lights. We are drawing on the analogy between the three colours of traffic signals and the range of mood swings a person may experience.

The green light is associated with the times when life is going well and mood swings are within an acceptable range. The amber light is associated with an increase in the severity of mood swings, and an urgent need to take steps to limit this increase. Life is becoming difficult. The red light is associated with danger, in our case an uncontrolled mood swing and its consequences. Life has become impossible and we are no longer in control. The aim of the course is to enable people to learn to keep the lights at green as much as possible.

To date, over 160 men and women with manic depression have completed the programme. Early findings reveal that although participants on the programme are generally very positive about self-management, they lack confidence in the current mental health system. Our research shows that it takes on average ten years to make an accurate diagnosis of manic depression. Participants feel community psychiatric nurses and counsellors do not understand the illness. Almost two-thirds of the participants were either 'positive' or 'very positive' about the medication they were taking, but they did have concerns about its long-term side-effects.

Suicide rates for manic depression are higher than for other psychiatric risk groups, and it is extremely positive that participants on the self-management training programme experience fewer suicidal thoughts or wishes after they have completed the programme. This finding sends a clear message to the mental health system and policy-making bodies that self-management adds an important dimension to conventional methods of treatment.

Many members of the Manic Depression Fellowship with a diagnosis of manic depression are finding that a good quality of life is usually possible with effective self-management. Here are a selection of comments made by participants:

'I feel more in control of my psychiatrist, he found that my advanced directive was the highest level of insight he had ever come across in a patient'

'It's spring, I'm normally in hospital now'

'Everyone had some constructive input to make and it was wonderful to be able to draw upon the combined wealth of experience of the participants. There was a common purpose – to keep well and get well'

Through a user-led approach the Manic Depression Fellowship is enabling individuals to become empowered and take control over their own lives, which in turn appears to be leading to greater social inclusion.

A double life: a selective autobiography

Anonymous

Life as a child was happy and secure, but I may have acquired a psychological vulnerability to depression during my first decade. My mother recently reminded me of her own teenage depression, when she moved from under the umbrella of school into the world of work.

Our family moved around the country as my father's career progressed. I was put up a year at school at the age of seven, which I took completely in my stride at the time, soon rising to the top of my new class. I attended four schools up to secondary level. It was hard to make and keep friends, or to learn social confidence, but safe in the bosom of the family I was happily unaware of this.

At the age of twelve I moved into a class of thirteen-going-on-fourteen year olds, all of whom seemed to be interested in horses, clothes, pop music or boys, none of which ever appealed to me as a teenager (going into a pub, let alone listening to pop music or fancying boys, seemed to approximate to depravity in my parents' eyes).

I became socially withdrawn. I used to walk from class to class with my nose buried in a book. I had periods that I characterised to myself as my grey days and I knew I wasn't happy. At the age of fifteen I had a nice collection of mosses and liverworts, but no friends.

The sixth form at a new school was a happy time, but not long enough to allow me to complete my developmental tasks. To my amazement I was offered a place to read Natural Sciences at Cambridge. I had never been away from home for more than a few days until then and homesickness set in rapidly.

I can't remember how my difficulties were picked up. An appointment with the university counselling service was arranged for me, and I also acquired some antidepressants via my new GP. The chaplain and his family offered support. At the appointed hour I slunk fearfully to the counselling service building, scanning the street to ensure there were no familiar faces (some chance). To my horror, the counsellor's verdict was that I should see a psychiatrist within the week. I was overcome with shame and inadequacy. I knew nothing of depression or mental illness.

I yielded to the overwhelming yearning to seek refuge at the chaplain's house for a little while – an open invitation I had been careful never to take up. I needed people. When the door was opened I dissolved into wordless, silent sobs.

I was moved immediately to the chaplain's home and soon gave up all pretence of work. What's it like, seeing a psychiatrist for the first time? For many people this would be akin to a major life event, something to be faced with trepidation, but by then I was so far withdrawn inwardly that I don't retrospectively associate any fear or anxiety with the event.

On the way back from the second appointment the psychiatrist phoned to say that I should be admitted to some sort of psychiatric unit in the town. By the time I got back to the chaplain's house, my bag had been packed and I was expected to go.

In fact I stayed only two nights, because the next day my tutor phoned my parents who collected me, and so I returned to Sheffield.

The lack of follow-up was disastrous. I would like to think it would not happen today. I should have transferred to the student health services in Sheffield, but my elderly GP referred me as a private patient to an adult psychiatrist. Two months after my return, I had a job as a laboratory technician at Bassett's Liquorice Allsorts, deep in working class Sheffield. I took a long time to settle. The other women realised how scared I was and generously provided a fair amount of mothering. I learned as much about life from Bassett's as I did at Cambridge and am grateful for the acceptance and friendship I found there.

The evening before I went back to college again, I sat on my mother's knee and wept. She even said I didn't have to go if I didn't want to, but I said I must.

This time I stayed the course. I saw the psychiatrist every week for what would be termed supportive psychotherapy for the three undergraduate years. I had a brief, inadequate trial of antidepressants; stopping them after my mother caught sight of the tablet bottle in my room. I signed up to do a PhD on river snails in Cambridge and I changed to one of the three graduate colleges. I no longer saw the psychiatrist, discovered men and gradually grew up. For the first time I started to question seriously what I was going to do with my life and a chance meeting set me exploring the path of medicine.

I lived in an eccentric but wonderful mixed house (in which I met my husband-to-be just before finals) and was altogether purposeful and happy.

In 1985, within six months, there were three major life events, four if the onset of a further depressive illness is included. Paradoxically this last came first, my fiancée recognising changes during a skiing holiday in January. In February we started living together for the first time in our own house in another city, and I became a senior house officer in psychiatry. In June we got married. I didn't feel recovered from the depression until October. Again, this episode was unreported and untreated, although not unrecognised at work, but as usual it was too little, too late. No one knew my pre-morbid self – another occupational hazard for the mobile junior doctor. I felt weak and ashamed to be depressed again, particularly having knowingly gone into the job, and just tried not to draw attention to myself.

I had met my psychiatrist socially on my return to Cambridge. She was delighted to see me and hugged me on hearing that I was coming back to do medicine. We remain in touch, and on occasion I have sounded out her opinion on relevant matters. As I recall, our conclusion concerning my application for a junior psychiatry post was to try it and see – fair enough.

Life events in 1987 clustered thick and fact. February: move to London, start registrar jobs, twin pregnancy. May: final specialist exams for both. I pass, he failed. June: the first routine ultrasound scan reveals the twins. Elation followed by a sense of immense fatigue sweeps over me, grandparents to be (first time on both sides) rhapsodic. July: depressed, I weep in front of the GP at an antenatal check, I am signed off for eight weeks before my maternity leave starts – but no further intervention. August: and I am in the psychiatrist's chair literally when I go to see our Professor, Anthony Clare, to ask for his support in my application for part-time senior registrar training. Halfway through he suddenly leans forward and says 'You look strained... how *are* you?' Like others before and since, he commented that I was totally different from my usual self, and on hearing that this had happened before, advised me to get myself referred to a psychiatrist (impressive: acute and effective). November: the twins are born, at almost forty weeks.

1988 by comparison was tranquil. I started working five sessions a week as a senior registrar from October 1988.

I discovered I was pregnant again in April 1989: three sons in two years. The twins were still in nappies.

Three months later I got depressed. This time I was started on amitriptyline, which worked. I didn't have time off, and started my maternity leave at thirty-eight weeks. I remember cycling up to the Angel Islington without stopping in the forty-first week of pregnancy. I was always in a hurry. Was I high? I took no notice of the first contractions and had just bathed the twins a few hours later when my waters broke.

After the birth I went back to the psychiatrist, with relief. She saw me weekly, but, even so, it was hard to keep going. If I could somehow make it to the watershed of about 3.00 pm, the rest of the day was relatively tolerable. But then the clouds came down.

I knew the psychiatrist would be away for several weeks in the summer holidays. At the penultimate appointment, the word admission was mentioned, in the context of brief respite, a last resort.

Two days later in August 1990, I was admitted to the acute psychiatric unit at a London teaching hospital under the care of a different psychiatrist. I was discharged almost six months later.

Depression is a common and severe disorder, with serious consequences for the individual, those around him or her and wider society. Women are twice as likely to suffer from depression as men. Depressive symptoms may be more common in disadvantaged people, but depression can affect people from all sections of society, including the health professions. This account of lifelong episodic depression describes the damaging effects of depression on the education, career and relationships of a young woman, training to be a doctor. It also provides a remarkable account of resilience to adversity, of how the effects of depression can be reduced and sometimes overcome.

Depression causes major personal turmoil and reduces quality of life. It can contribute to the breakdown of marriages and families, and in depressed mothers may sometimes delay the development of their children. It is difficult to comment on the health of someone without having met her, but in this account the author appears to describe the 'classical' symptoms of depression.

Depression has many causes, ranging from genetic predisposition to the effects of childhood trauma. Among other causative factors, the author describes the history of depression in her mother, the adverse effects of moving house on her childhood friendships and the untoward effects of high academic expectation. Most people believe that pregnancy and childbirth should be times of contented fulfillment, but she gives an unblinkered account of depressive episodes arising during pregnancy and after delivery – times in which depressive symptoms are actually rather common. She also describes the difficulties of mothering three young children, while simultaneously attempting to progress through her medical career. These causes can be counterbalanced by factors that act to increase personal resilience, and she also gives a clear account of the beneficial and protective effects of shared student accommodation, supportive intimate relationships and paid employment.

Once established, depression usually recurs and sometimes seems to develop a life of its own, independent of good or bad circumstances, beneficial or disruptive life changes. In this account, prolonged periods

COMMENTARY – DAVID BALDWIN

of comparative personal well-being are interrupted by frequent relapses into depression. It is uncertain whether the lack of continuity of medical care for the author after discharge from hospital, or the interruption of treatment during the postnatal depressive episode, might have increased her risk of relapsing, but psychiatrists try to minimise these discontinuities in medical care, in the belief that they are damaging and sometimes hazardous. When considering the course of her illness, she reflects on whether she may have experienced a brief period of abnormally elated mood (hypomanic episodes). On close questioning, many patients with recurring depression describe such episodes, which can lead to a revised diagnosis, and a different treatment emphasis, with the use of mood-stabilising drugs, and avoidance of certain antidepressants.

Stigma and discrimination make people who might be suffering from depression reluctant to seek treatment, and the recognition and treatment of depression by doctors and other health professionals can be poor. The author reports the difficulty in disclosing her health problems to even presumably sympathetic work colleagues.

This account describes the effects of recurring depression in a professional, married mother. How would a man have coped, if affected by this recurring and unpredictable condition? Although there is considerable overlap in the types of depressive symptoms experienced by men or women, male depression is rather more associated with restlessness, irritability and aggression, alcohol consumption and 'workaholism'. These behavioural manifestations of depression in men can lead to friction with partners and work colleagues, resulting in marital breakdown and unemployment. Men are at greater risk of suicide, but are less likely than women to present for help, or have their underlying depression recognised, and are also less likely to persist with treatment.

Depression is nasty and brutish, but not short. Most patients will experience recurring episodes of illness, but with treatment these can be shortened and many can be prevented. Public attitudes to depression have altered over the past decade, but more work is required to reduce misunderstanding and prejudice.

Depression and alcohol

Anonymous

In my childhood, I experienced a great deal of anxiety and depression but I did not have a name for these experiences. I was born the middle child of nine children to an alcoholic father and a mother who gambled and suffered from depression herself.

Because of suffering physical, mental, emotional and spiritual abuse, I began to run away from home at the early age of nine. I was detained in remand homes, approved schools, and borstal training institutes, going on to a young offenders institute by the age of seventeen. I had begun to shoplift from the age of about six, to provide basic needs for myself and my family. This was encouraged and so became a way of life for me. I began to self-harm when I was twelve or thirteen. The only acknowledgment of my problems was when I was treated with chlorpromazine at the age of thirteen and I was told this was because I was high spirited.

I experienced suicidal feelings when I was about fifteen and the GP referred me to a psychiatric unit in my home-town of Glasgow. After a short time there I was transferred to a larger hospital and detained in a locked ward, owing to self-harming behaviour. Within a week, I was discharged. My next admission to a psychiatric unit was after the death of my younger brother, when I made a suicide attempt at the borstal institution. I remained in that unit for six weeks and received no medication or therapy.

When I was nineteen and training to be a nurse, I once again felt suicidal and took my first overdose. This occurred on numerous further occasions and I was diagnosed as being a psychopath but offered no help in dealing with my problems. All I understood from this diagnosis was that I was some kind of murderer and feared the day I would indeed murder someone. It meant to me that I was someone without feelings and I felt very mixed up about it because I knew that I did have feelings.

It was inevitable that I was attracted into a very dysfunctional relationship with a man and had a child with him. He was an alcoholic and, about that time, I began to drink heavily too. I suffered much abuse within this relationship and finally left after three years in fear that my child would also suffer if I stayed. I continued to drink heavily every night.

At twenty-four, I married into another dysfunctional relationship and had four more children, as well as two miscarriages and a second abortion. I had stopped self-harming and was able to raise my children for a number of years, though still drinking every night.

As my drinking worsened, I began to experience the trauma of delirium tremens, whenever I tried to stop drinking. Shaking, violent sweating, vomiting and terrible fears were common symptoms to me. Hangovers made daily functioning difficult, sometimes impossible.

I was not aware that I was an alcoholic, even though all of my family, except for my mother, were. In 1986, when my father died, I began to question myself about my drinking. I saw my GP, who referred me to a consultant psychiatrist specialising in alcoholism. He asked about my drinking and told me that I was severely depressed.

Although about that time I joined a fellowship, which used the twelve-step programme, in the hope of dealing with my drinking problem, I ignored the consultant's advice about my being severely depressed because I did not believe this to be true.

Unable to stop drinking for more than a few months at a time, I finally began to feel the full force of my illness in 1991. I could no longer cope with life as I had been doing. I felt that I was unable to go on for another day. It was at this point that I took myself back to the consultant and asked for help. I was sectioned under the Mental Health Act because I felt suicidal. It was explained to me that I was severely depressed but I still found that hard to believe. After spending five months in the hospital, I began to realise that the way I was feeling was known as depression. I could see no reason to live, I had lost any sense of feeling that I had had before. More importantly to me, I no longer cared about my life or my children. Everything seemed pointless and I had no motivation left for anything. Food became increasingly difficult to eat. Sometimes I would only eat at the insistence of others.

From that day to this I have had a great struggle to stop drinking. It is now just over one year since I wanted to drink alcohol, the longest I've ever been without it. My marriage ended and I now live alone with my children. Self-harming and suicidal thoughts and attempts have been a pattern of behaviour for me since I was first admitted to hospital in 1991.

I experience depression of varying degrees, which does not respond very well to antidepressants. I suffer nightmares, and often find it difficult to get through the day. I have little appetite and my sleep is poor. I take sleeping medication.

Last year I spent some time working with a clinical psychologist. I am now in the process of being assessed to receive treatment in the form of intensive group psychotherapy.

The author's description of her struggles against depression and addiction makes disturbing reading and she gives a moving account of both childhood deprivation and the difficulties that often accompany it. Unfortunately the pattern she describes is not uncommon, especially where, as in her case, her father was alcoholic and her mother depressed. Children of alcoholics have more than their share of insecurity, and if the other parent is depressed this doubles the problem. Rutter and Smith (1995) have emphasised the influences of family and environment in causing difficulties for children in their development.

Added to this is the effect of institutions. In trying to escape from an abusive home, she found herself detained in the often impersonal environment of the juvenile offenders' system. Her low self-esteem, self-harm and suicidal feelings are all too understandable in the light of these earlier experiences.

People who have experienced this kind of childhood may develop many different patterns of disturbance. In this case it has been mainly depression, self-harm and alcoholism, but in other cases bulimia, drug misuse or psychosis may occur, and the suicide rate is higher than in the rest of the population. Relationships are particularly difficult, and in some people relationships are impossible because of the complete inability to trust an intimate partner. She describes her first relationship as abusive and her second as dysfunctional. The second lasted considerably longer, and may have been viable only for as long as she was drinking (in itself a dysfunctional factor). It may be significant that this marriage ended when she gave up alcohol.

Taking control of her life was a very important step forward, and the joining of the twelve-step programme seems to have begun to break the cycle of drinking and lack of control, and given her time to think.

In the past year, with abstinence from alcohol and help from the clinical psychologist, she appears to have made real progress. The proposed group psychotherapy is again a hopeful factor, and will help her if she can get it. Although she says the antidepressants do not help very much, they seem to be having some impact on her depression, and it may be that without them she would feel more distress.

She is a survivor in the best sense of the word, and she has done well to have a marriage that lasted some years, and to be able to raise her family of five children. She is clearly more vulnerable than most people, and future stress could lead to depression or a relapse into alcoholism. However, she has considerable strengths, and has survived many past stresses without collapsing, and with support and help she may well remain stable and free of addiction.

On my unit at the Bethlem Royal Hospital, dealing specifically with people who self-harm, we see many patients, both male and female, who have had negative childhood experiences and whose current pattern of behaviour includes self-harm, suicidal attempts, bulimia, drug and alcohol misuse, low self-esteem, self-hatred, depression and relationship problems (Crowe & Bunclark, 2000). This is a group of patients who up to now have had less help than other general psychiatric patients, although their problems of adjustment may be just as great. Motivational difficulties and ambivalence towards treatment make them 'difficult to help', and their need for a dependent relationship can make it sometimes problematic to treat them in psychotherapy.

There are, however, some hopeful signs, and these include the development of some effective treatment approaches, such as dialectical behavioural therapy (Linehan, 1993), cognitive therapy (Salkovskis *et al*, 1990) and the use of 'emergency cards' for accident and emergency attendance. Community health teams are developing strategies to help abuse survivors and self-harmers, and family therapy can help both the patients and their partners and children to understand the problems and cope with them.

In those who have suffered sexual abuse, it is probably best not to go into too much detail in therapy, but preferable to 'reclaim the self' and to work on self-esteem in the here and now (Crowe & Dare, 1998).

So, although nothing can be done to change the past, survivors of all kinds of childhood abuse can often overcome the after-effects and live more healthy and satisfying lives with the help of therapy.

It was seventeenth June 1999. I was in Dublin and I'd just missed the band I'd been sent to review for a magazine. I was drunk and stoned, as I had been for some weeks. Friends were worried. Apparently I'd been talking to my computer and it had been talking back. But as far as I was concerned life was cool. I'd split up with an alcoholic double my age and he'd stopped berating me on the mobile phone thirty times a day. My work as a journalist and as a DJ was in recovery and I was in Dublin.

Although I did not know it, I was acting strangely. Drawing postcards at the bar, proudly emptying my Gucci handbag of its contents, lining up the cosmetics for all to view. More people than usual asked me if I had any drugs to sell. In the morning I took a cab to the airport. I lost an unrequired passport and my ticket. They wouldn't let me on the plane. I thought I had to save the world, I ran between the bureau de change and the departure board tallying up random numbers from departures and writing them down on bureau de change slips.

When this didn't work I began to pick up bits of rubbish from the floor; I thought they were clues left for me by the London art underworld. I thought I was a living sculpture/installation and started a performance next to the security desk. The police arrived and took me for questioning. Before long I was in an ambulance. At the hospital I thought I was doing a royal visit and mistook the admission form for a death certificate. Excellent, I thought, only I could get away with a fake death.

Having gone to look for a smoking room I fell on an exit and left. I walked for a few hours and found my way back to Dublin. There I made enquiries about my passport. Nothing. Later I met a guy in a funny suit, Brian. We went for a milkshake. He turned out to be rotten, weird and full of lies. Over the next week, like a magpie he had taken my jewellery and my clothes.

He persuaded me to stay in Ireland for the summer solstice. I thought it might make a good story. He'd told me of some parties happening and to be honest it sounded like a good break. My life had been hectic for a long time. He'd told me he was a singer, and I said I'd manage him.

So together, armed with staffs made from sticks and lumps of amethyst, we roamed the countryside, often getting in trouble. One night I found myself in a jacuzzi, the next I'd be in a farmer's bed. We'd get thrown out

Drug-induced psychosis

Randy Osqviff

of pubs because, unknown to me, Brian had been there before. Walking all night, surviving on Guinness, became a bit much so we returned to the city. Here I lost Brian; he'd been doing my head in with his pseudo-healing and crap singing. I picked up men who looked after me and enjoyed the madness. I developed theories about the Liffey being the centre force and thought a film was being made about me. I was constantly being hurled out of pubs and bars; in London I'd always been able to get in anywhere. By this time I'd lost all my possessions. One night I walked along a canal, another I watched cranes and workmen. One time I was in a club and a girl gave me an E. When the club finished I lost the wanton men and found a squat party, I DJ-ed and tidied up when it was over. In the morning I went for coffee and had a go at shoplifting, then gave the trinkets to a bunch of kids who followed me for a while. I walked through the suburbs picking flowers from every garden, believing them to contain healing powers. An Oasis fan came out of his house and asked if I wanted to go in for coffee. Just as my new friend had asked a police car pulled up. Apparently there'd been a few phone calls. They sat me down for a cup of tea at the station. This was the fourth time I'd been in a police station all week. They took me to a hospital. I was put out.

I don't remember arriving at St Brendan's psychiatric ward. It was a sad place for about fourteen women. I tried to escape once but failed. I made one friend. My dad flew over immediately; my mum followed a week later. My main concern was getting back to my home in London's Clerkenwell. I was helping to organise a street festival. It took another week and a half to get out of St Brendan's. People rang me, including the ex. He'd just written a book and dedicated it to me, which added to the stress.

I was transferred to Ealing Hospital's John Connolly Ward. I was there for five weeks. I saw people slit their wrists and fights, but generally it was OK. After that I moved back to my parents' house, where I still am.

I'm better now. I came off the haloperidol at Christmas. I'm in drugs counselling and I don't go out every night. I've been temping a bit but I hope to get back into writing. The depression after hospital was horrendous; the side-effects of the drugs were also intolerable. I'm thinking about training as a mental health worker.

Problems with drugs and alcohol

Keith Murray

Born in 1952, third of five boys. Father, Bernard, studied chemistry before wartime RAF then civil aviation as pilot. Mother, Fioni Llewellyn, dancing and elocution teacher before wartime WRAF then housewife.

Family moved from West Drayton to Scotland when I was five, following Dad's job. Here I went to local schools, doing very well until senior secondary. I began failing exams and losing interest. I hated Greenock High from day one.

By age sixteen I occasionally had a drink, filched from parents' sitting room. Regularly smoking too. First pubs around seventeen – very convivial.

Mum was warm and comforting, but no pushover. Dad was strict and I was mainly afraid of him. He was kind, too. His punishments were severe, but rarely physical. His work took him away from home for several days at a time, and I usually dreaded him coming home.

I left home at eighteen with six O-Levels and a Higher in English, Dad having found me a temporary job and digs in London.

In my twenties, my social life revolved around pubs or parties. The latter always made me nervous and I would usually drink excessively.

I never settled. I shared flats with friends – successfully at first. I worked as a van driver, labourer, arborist (I enjoyed that particularly) and in 1979 began fourteen years as a motorcycle messenger.

Age twenty-one I tried marijuana. By twenty-five I was smoking it daily and protecting my supply. This habit continued until 1996. I tried other drugs, that is LSD, cocaine and speed. Of these I liked LSD and used it periodically, but not frequently until around 1993.

Looking back, I was in some kind of trouble by 1980. Around then I stopped going to parties. I was getting what I now think were panic attacks – no breathlessness but a very sudden, deep feeling of fear, inadequacy, uselessness right in the middle of a party or pub gathering, usually when there were many people around. Around this time I started drinking at home, with or without company. I was working only enough hours to pay the rent and drink and drug bills – two to three days a week.

In 1980 I was supposed to be saving for the 'trip of a lifetime', a year's working holiday in Australia, but I was too lethargic to earn enough even for the ticket. Eventually, my brother Patrick, who lived in Tasmania, bought it and I went out in 1981 with my leaving pay packet and ninety pounds for the bike.

I worked hard as a driller's mate but I found myself alone at weekends and drank heavily.

After six months I was able to leave Tasmania with enough money to buy a car. I went to Southport, New South Wales, to meet a co-worker from the drilling job.

Eventually, I started work as a wood-chipping plant operator in Brisbane. I learned that being in a different country did not change my attitudes. I was still unmotivated, and if there were any problems with the machinery I would make little effort to get it going but simply close down the shift and go home.

I returned from Australia in late 1982 and got back to work as a courier. I lived with a friend near Bermondsey. In March 1983 I got into trouble with a pub landlord who, after much provocation, bashed me with a cut-down cue, causing the loss of my left eye. Drink was involved, in that I wouldn't have been so loud-mouthed without it.

It didn't occur to me, even after the 'eye' incident, that I had a drink problem. Depression, sure. Anxiety, perhaps.

A year after losing my eye I was back to work on bikes but nothing much had changed. I shared flats with people but I was morose unless drinking and not good company. I was asked to move on a few times. I fell back into working only sufficient time to maintain my minimum lifestyle of cigarettes, drink and marijuana. I began to 'get into' computer games – my fourth drug, as I came to think of it later. Where I had no (nor any longer sought) relationships, the interactive screen became substitute.

Following a letter to my parents, I was introduced to the Tavistock Clinic for Human Relations.

Around 1987 I went to the weekly group for two years and found it a waste of time. I was living near Beckenham at the time. I got beaten up at a party about a mile from home, which is where I found myself the next morning, bruised, bloody and with no recollection of what had happened. I discovered later that I'd upset an ex-para. I decided to take three months away from alcohol, just to make sure that I could. I did.

I moved a couple more times, winding up in a bedsit in Streatham, a slightly dingy, damp place, but it was mine; I paid the rent and felt secure for the first time in years. At first, I used the (very) local pub, but they took away the pin-table and pool table. This also took away my people-buffers so I stopped going. I was in a cycle of drink, dope, work and computer games, which never really ended until I got to rehab in January 1996.

As my fortieth birthday approached (9th January, 1992), I decided that my present to myself and my family would be to take a year away from alcohol. Although I didn't think that it was my primary problem, it sure was something I needed to look at. I cut out dope at the same time, but that only lasted three weeks. I wasn't particularly aware of any changes. I still wasn't going out unless I had to, although I would very occasionally meet an old friend in a pub; I'd drink tonic or coke.

I bought a car, an old banger, early in this 'dry' period. The idea was that, because one of my excuses for not visiting folk was dodgy weather and my growing fear of death by motorcycle, the car would give me freedom. I took it on a trip to Scotland, visiting relatives, but only used it twice more in London. I just didn't like going out.

In October, I promised myself that I could have a drink the following New Year's Eve, which I duly did, very moderately. I then waited the remaining nine days before letting myself see if I could drink 'like a gentleman'. Within a month I was back in the same old pattern. I went to see my GP about what turned out to be thrush. I asked for a psychiatric assessment. He suspected diabetes and sent me to hospital for tests.

I persisted with requests for a psychiatric assessment and was eventually referred. I paid myself to take ten weeks off work to attend the Drink Crisis Centre four days a week, where I learned a great deal about the mechanics of alcohol abuse, but didn't apply the lifestyle information provided. I also went to one-to-one counselling, which I didn't find of any use.

In April 1994 I left work. I was so distracted with my 'problems' all the time that I was convinced I'd have an accident. Probably would have. I left work with a clean license. The psychiatrist referred me to the Addiction Clinic to stop smoking, which I did for eighteen months, only taking it up again when I was admitted to hospital for a six-week detox. While there, I had my first meaningful contact with AA.

I went to have ten months of rehabilitation. I liked the groups and didn't mind the numbers of people and general mayhem too much. I had to go to at least three AA meetings a week and frequently went to more. I went to an open learning centre and taught myself to use Microsoft programs such as Word, Access and Excel. I became a volunteer assistant trainer and stayed with the open learning centre for some time.

The rehabilitation staff were true to their word and found me my current flat, in Battersea. I took the plunge into the world of work again. This period was a time of hope. I never missed the alcohol or dope. I learned much about myself and people in general. In January 1998 I took the job of IT tutor with the group who ran the open learning centre, knowing that I would be virtually no better off financially, but believing that it would lead to better things.

I became disaffected at work – I didn't see eye-to-eye with my immediate boss and hated the commercial aspects of the job. I became depressed again. By May I was smoking dope and by June was drinking. I hung onto the job until September, when our section was closed down. I went back into hospital, stopped drinking and attended a day group three times a week. In January I drank again and had to leave. I've been muddling along since then.

COMMENTARY

– EMILY FINCH

These very personal and honest accounts by two people whose lives have been radically changed by their use of different substances are fascinating reading. They are a timely reminder to me and I hope to anyone who reads them of aspects of substance use disorders that are easy to forget.

In the treatment services where I work there is often a conspiracy between many of the service users, the doctors, nurses and others who try to help them and (possibly crucially) those who plan and pay for the services. This conspiracy is that substance misuse problems are easy to treat and that the individuals' problems are somehow trivial. The substance users themselves believe this because they genuinely want to be better and want to have a problem that can be solved after a few months of treatment. After all who wouldn't? The individuals who provide treatment want their treatments to work quickly and well. They may confuse harm reduction interventions such as the provision of clean needles and quick detoxification treatments with a permanent cure. The harm reduction interventions are valuable and needed but they must not be confused with the complex and long-term process of achieving permanent abstinence. The system that plans and pays for services wants to provide interventions that are cost-effective and wants brief treatments to work well.

Long-term or intensive interventions are expensive and difficult to deliver. The account of the way alcohol has dominated Keith's life should persuade us all to accept what a long-term and severe problem an addiction can be. Probably the only treatment philosophy that completely accepts this is the alcoholics and narcotics anonymous one. As an approach it has many critics and faults but its acknowledgement of the long-term nature of addiction needs hearing.

These accounts of lives changed by substance misuse are profoundly personal. They demonstrate how addiction problems penetrate to the deepest regions of an individual's inner experience and to their contacts with the outside world, their work, their relationships and their identity. Randy's account of her drug-induced psychotic illness and the changes it induced in her personality and behaviour illustrates this graphically.

The process people have to drag themselves through to overcome these problems is an enormous one.

The link between these accounts is the use of substances. In other ways they offer very different experiences of the problems. Substance misuse may present people with a variety of problems from acute periods of psychiatric illness as illustrated by Randy's account or the long daily grind of alcohol dependence as illustrated by Keith's.

Neither account says much about the treatment system. Detoxification or an in-patient admission is a small part of the experience of the illness. Doctors, nurses and drug workers can, arrogantly, believe that their intervention in the life of an addicted individual is the most important one. We all forget people's daily struggle with their illness, which goes on when they are not in the clinic or on the ward. Even detoxification, which appears a defining event in the course of an illness while it is happening, may seem trivial in the life of an individual living with an addiction problem.

Treatment is only a small part of the experience of an individual struggling to become and remain abstinent from drugs. Almost all of the work is done by those individuals themselves. They resist or succumb to cravings, deal with daily withdrawal symptoms and learn to understand the triggers that make them relapse. Many deal with disabling psychiatric symptoms that accompany their misuse of substances. At its best, treatment must enhance substance users' own strengths and enable them to use their own abilities to support their recovery. It is about providing people with psychological and pharmacological tools that they can put to good effect. Plainly, we are unable to solve their problems for them.

Perhaps the most important lesson to gain from these accounts is to listen to our patients. They grow to know and understand their addictions better than us and can usually tell us how to plan their care. We can learn how to develop services more sensitively so that they will be appropriate to users at different stages in the course of their illness. Our patients will also remind us to be humble and to acknowledge the huge power and pervasiveness of addiction.

Living with obsessive–compulsive disorder

Daisy Fields

My contribution to this book is a big secret – because I work in a psychological field directly with patients and, unknown to my employers or my friends, I have an obsessive–compulsive disorder (OCD). Only my partner knows about my condition.

In OCD the sufferer experiences anxiety – often very severe – caused by irrational intrusive thoughts ('obsessions') that he or she is driven to allay through the performance of rituals ('compulsions').

OCD and me

I had a strict Catholic home-life, and was a boarder at convent school from the age of seven. In those days (and I am 'mature' now) convents really were severe. My OCD has a strong moral/religious tinge, with powerful feelings of guilt and shame, which, though I am no longer a Catholic, I'm sure have come from that influence.

From about aged eight, I developed worries with rituals. All of these, or their remnants, have remained or spasmodically returned over the years, and I've never been really free of them. Mainly, these were: first, at eight, a terrible fear of leaving the attic light on at home and harming my parents by wasting their money; so I kept climbing up to re-check; from about nine, a terror of committing a mortal sin – for which, we were taught, I would go to hell for eternity unless I got it forgiven before I died (which could be at any moment); also around nine, a 'Lady Macbeth' need to wash my hands and body excessively, one of my most persistent problems; and at about fourteen fears around sex. I knew virtually nothing about sex, and had understood from our teacher that the slightest momentary sexual thought was a mortal sin. That single statement terrified me, and was the only Catholic teaching on sex that I received at school. I also had a horror of toilets – with long phases of avoiding public toilets altogether, reducing my work and social opportunities; a fear of hurting others through poisons or chemicals, or bits of food that had gone bad; a dread of harming anyone by what I might say or write. In my profession, this has entailed my spending extra time (unpaid) in re-checking my own written work.

As a child I tried to ask some grown-ups for help about these things, but they did not understand and I felt so ashamed that I stopped telling anyone ever again.

What interventions have helped and what have not?

As a young student, I cracked-up. I could not stop washing and I found myself in an old, asylum-type mental hospital as a voluntary patient. Medication was then crude, and ECT ruled (although I never had it). I was the only OCD patient, and received 'chats' plus intensive chlorpromazine, which confined me to bed, with boils, sleepiness and the shakes – but no improvement. I stayed for eight months. The memories of that place won't leave me, and have become more of my shameful secrets.

After that, I tried various therapies, for example I spent twelve years under a Freudian psychoanalyst, without success.

Eventually, in 1989, I embarked on behavioural therapy in which people with OCD undergo intensive, repeated 'exposure' to their feared situations without performing rituals, until their anxiety becomes negligible. This comprised my being an NHS in-patient at a specialist unit, a luxurious environment compared with my asylum experience of many years before. But the regime was purely behavioural, harshly ignoring patients' feelings and thoughts. Nevertheless, after nine weeks I left, greatly improved.

However, ten years later, following a stressful period, I relapsed. Seemingly, behavioural therapy trains our will to stop doing rituals, but it doesn't necessarily cure the residual irrational belief in the need to do them.

Then I discovered BTSTEPS (a telephone based system of behavioural therapy for OCD), provided by therapists from the same unit in London, on the NHS and with no admission to hospital. It also includes cognitive therapy (which works with the thoughts/beliefs) if needed to reduce residual irrational beliefs.

The availability of the BTSTEPS' telephone therapist especially helped me. My first therapist, assisted administratively by his wife, was warm, accepting and so good for my self-esteem that I have, for example, resumed much more ambitious professional work. Later, a different therapist helped my beliefs through cognitive therapy. An excellent course that improved me greatly.

Very recently I have been severely ill physically. Following that, my OCD has partially worsened again. Maybe a further BTSTEPS course is on my horizon.

Conclusion

For me, the worst part of OCD is the secrecy. I hide my illness, for work and social reasons. So, apart from my partner (God bless him), I avoid close friendships as I can't be open in them.

From my experience, behavioural plus cognitive therapies seem currently the best OCD treatment, but they don't cure it. They merely make the fears manageable, through an ongoing effort of will (and courage) on the behaviour and thoughts. Any let-up can produce a relapse. But today there is help.

Daisy's account illustrates important aspects of OCD and how current self-help methods can help individuals to overcome the problems without ever having to see a therapist face-to-face. Her most recent (and successful) self-treatment was guided mostly by a computer system called BTSTEPS, from which she sought advice at intervals, accessing the computer by phoning from home (BT refers to behaviour therapy, not a UK phone company). More on that later.

The first point Daisy makes is how important she has found it since childhood to keep her OCD secret from friends and employers, so only her partner knows about her problem. She says she feels she must conceal her difficulties because she works with patients in a psychological field. Such shame is a major issue for people who have OCD or other mental health problems. It explains why most people with anxiety and depressive disorders who are identified in the community do not get treatment for their problem. Many employers look askance at job applicants who have a mental health record, and a record of that kind could sound the death knell for a political career. Reporters ferret around searching for evidence of 'instability' with which to damn candidates, though in fact mild OCD is perfectly compatible with making an excellent contribution to public life.

Daisy had been distressed by her OCD for decades before she sought help using behavioural psychotherapy. More public discussion about OCD and other anxiety disorders would reduce the stigma associated with them and encourage people to come for help earlier. Getting effective help early reduces the seriousness of the illness.

The dreaded worries that Daisy writes about so vividly are typical of OCD. Her thoughts revolved around themes of harming others or herself unless she carried out particular rituals, including checking and washing, and avoided contaminating situations and substances. Also classic was the severity of Daisy's problem – hours of washing and repeated in-patient admissions. Fortunately she managed to continue working and to have a partner. Many sufferers lose their jobs and families owing to OCD. They may spend much of their days and nights engaged in endless and pointless washing and/or checking, or just sitting in a chair immobile because getting up from there would start hours of interminable rituals, and they would be unable to do anything else.

Daisy describes past abortive attempts at treatment, including medication and twelve years of 'Freudian psychoanalysis' until she finally improved for ten years after nine weeks of behaviour therapy as an in-patient. Even today many healthcare professionals, even those in the mental health field, do not know that for thirty years OCD has been treated successfully by the form of behaviour therapy called 'exposure plus ritual prevention', and that in the past few years self-treatment (by self-exposure and self-imposed ritual prevention) has been effective with minimal input from a professional.

BTSTEPS

Daisy's experience with BTSTEPS needs further explanation. She lived far from the specialist service and never saw a therapist face-to-face. The first therapist screened her in a phone interview to check that she could use BTSTEPS. Once found to be suitable, she was posted a self-help manual and an ID number to phone BTSTEP's computer-guidance system from the comfort of her home at any time of the day or night. By pressing keys on her telephone keypad she decided which of 800 different voice files of individually tailored advice the computer would play for her to hear.

A central observation of Daisy's is that she stays well by doing relapse prevention exercises involving exposure and ritual prevention homework – by facing things she would rather avoid and 'working on beliefs', meaning facing them and the feared consequences of doing so instead of avoiding them.

Daisy's experience shows that people with OCD can today treat themselves successfully without having to see a therapist face-to-face. They can self-treat from home by telephoning for brief advice from a live clinician and phoning for much longer guidance from an interactive-voice-response computer system such as BTSTEPS (see Organisations that can Help).

Growing up

Anonymous

I was happy as a kid. I don't remember it but I have been told it and can see it in the eyes of the little girl in our photo albums. Yet with hindsight, an obsessive personality was formed very early and the seeds of my anorexia sown at a preciously young age.

On my ninth birthday, I blamed myself for having a second slice of my favourite chocolate biscuit cake when I'd caught another sick bug. I remember the absolute terror of vomiting that gripped me. Away from home I wouldn't eat strangers' food.

I had problems sleeping too. By the age of nine or ten, I'd developed a belief that in any environment not entirely familiar to me, it was not safe to eat or sleep. Eating would make me physically sick and that was the worst thing that could happen to me.

I was a high achiever. Not only that, but in comparison with my naughty little sister, I was also the 'good girl' of the family, for which I earned praise, approval and pride. Being anorexic involves striving to achieve a state of purity and self-control that far exceeds what others do and pushes you to extreme limits. Paradoxically, in trying to be the supremely golden girl you accidentally make yourself the child from hell.

At the age of eight we moved house and I changed school, moving into a class of girls a year older than me. For the first year I was teased about being younger and brighter than the others, who in their jealousy taunted me that I smelt and picked my nose.

The greatest blow came when I was a year or so older and Mum became gradually ill with a chronic and debilitating neurological condition that crept up on the family and dealt us several years of trauma. The illness created an uncertain future in which she could at any time live or die. With Mum in and out of hospital, I took over the role of mother in the house and appeared to cope admirably with cooking, shopping, cleaning and washing, making sure that all was operating as normally as possible. In many ways I was being forced to grow up far ahead of my years and my resistance to that shows clearly in my anorexia, which was my way of 'growing down' at the same time.

I was managing to achieve near stability, through consistently undereating myself, and overeating under the supervision of Mum. I was able to go about school life apparently normally.

My hope was that I would go to university and fit in so well that weight issues simply vanished. However, already things were slipping out of anyone's control and I was obviously ill. I remember the horror of first seeing the sign on my psychiatrist's door and registering its significance. He helped me to work with my Mum to restore some weight so that I was in relatively good physical shape – although at seventeen I still had not undergone puberty. We acknowledged the trauma of Mum's illness and hoped that it was consigned to history and bundled me off.

It was an anorexic hell. I lasted just over a term. With regret but also relief I accepted time out and began a brief period of day care. With Mum's help the weight went back on, but in my head I had never really connected myself with the other girls I saw struggling to come to terms with weight-gain and fighting their illnesses. Family therapy proved disastrous and so Mum and Dad were not unhappy with the idea of my returning to university.

So I began again, but nothing had really changed. Indeed, if anything, my behaviour had become even further estranged from that of my fellow students. Somehow I managed to sit my first year exams and did remarkably well, but it was only a matter of time before I had to give up a second time.

My family's patience was wearing thin. My sister could no longer even bear to be in the same room as me and treated me with absolute contempt. Mum and Dad rowed about the control Mum tried to impose. It is with tremendous guilt that I recall all that I have put the family through.

Life at home was becoming unbearable for all. As my weight slipped away from me, Mum and Dad tried increasingly desperately to feed me and I rejected them more and more. I behaved like a frightened, wild animal and on several occasions threw platefuls of food around the kitchen, which had become our battleground. In desperation one day Mum and I sat in the waiting room of our GP's surgery and begged for a hospital bed for me.

I developed eating problems at the age of nineteen when I was at college. I do not intend to dwell on the various causal factors in detail, but suffice to say that during the summer of 1976 I went from being a happy teenager to a neurotic, socially withdrawn, desperately unhappy individual.

I had been weight training for four years, and had built up to around 12st 8lb. I was very strong and, although not all muscle, I certainly was not fat. I never really worried about food, except to eat fairly healthily, but basically ate whatever I wanted.

During the summer of 1976 I decided to loose some body fat as I had a desire to become really muscular. I did feel this pressure to be as attractive as possible to the opposite sex, and so I decided to follow a diet high in protein and low in carbohydrates.

Eating disorders in men

Anonymous

At the same time I 'upped' my training, and started to work out every day.

At first I felt much better; I could 'pose' in the mirror and see muscle fibres standing out to attention. My confidence increased and I drew admiring stares. I selected carefully, but was still fairly relaxed about food. However, after about six weeks I noticed that I no longer had this elated feeling. Instead I became more anxious. Every time I looked in the mirror, and saw this muscular body, I felt frightened of losing control and losing my 'new' body. I also increasingly dwelt on what food I had eaten or was about to eat. These thoughts permeated my waking day, and started to affect my behaviour.

At first I became distracted for odd moments. Gradually, however, as the anxiety took hold, these periods increased. I would sit in lectures (I was at teacher training college) and just couldn't concentrate. Lecturers would ask if I was OK. Of course I said yes. At this point I realised that my eating and training had become a problem.

Apart from this distraction element, I was becoming obsessive. I had to train. If I missed a workout I became desperately anxious and thought I would become fat again. I found that I shied away from social activities as they might make me miss a workout. I also became increasingly anxious about the food I was eating. I worried if I was forced to eat something different. I would sit at the table, trying to work out how many calories I was eating. Of course, while I was doing this, I took no part in conversation, and people, good friends, asked me if I felt OK – I did feel embarrassed and knew that what I was doing was making me unhappy, but felt completely unable to help myself. I believed this was the price to pay for a more muscular body.

On several occasions friends would invite me out, but I found these occasions very stressful, as I would agonise over menus and felt I was an embarrassment to the others there. I can remember virtually leaving meals if they came with butter or a sauce, or sending food back.

My increasingly bizarre behaviour around food led to me gradually withdrawing from social situations where food was involved. I spent an increasing amount of time on my own, and only then felt safe and in control. I preferred to eat alone. Although I was in a poor financial state, buying my own food was preferable to eating with others, with all the anxieties and problems it brought.

I did have a girlfriend, but saw very little of her. She obviously knew I was 'funny' about food, but never questioned me about it, apart from saying that 'all this training and dieting is making you boring'. I knew again that my behaviour and refusal to eat in public affected our relationship in that we never went out for a meal (except on very rare occasions and that led me to being stressed all day). Also, my preoccupation with food mentally and physically exhausted me – I had no energy for anything. I did play the guitar, but I found that this was merely a distraction to kill time between meals.

After six months I was in the grip of an eating disorder. I could only eat small amounts of food (although I still exercised obsessively) and spent all my time either on my own or, when I was in the company of others, I might just as well have been on my own. I became a food bore! All I would talk about was food, calories and exercise. I was unkind to people I felt didn't measure up to my idea of physical perfection. This was not me; I became another person, sullen and withdrawn. The only relief I got was either when I was asleep or when I was out running or weight-training. For a few moments I would be relaxed and able to think. However, sooner or later, all my anxieties about what to eat and how much would descend like a dark cloud.

Although I found socialising around food stressful, I also avoided going out with friends because I couldn't wear smart well-fitting clothes. I could only wear certain items of clothing that felt loose, nothing that hugged the body. The result was I looked like a tramp. Certainly I couldn't have made myself more unattractive.

After a year I was virtually a recluse, venturing out only to lectures or to train. People stopped asking me if I was OK – they stopped caring. Did they know I had an eating disorder? Probably, but this was the mid-1970s and most people would not have been familiar with eating problems.

My recovery took many years because I felt scared of admitting my problems to anyone, because of fear of being labelled 'mentally ill'. I found that most areas of my life had become ritualised, and breaking these compulsions (i.e., exercising or eating certain products) difficult and stressful. I did find certain activities such as playing the guitar, which boosted my self-esteem, helped, and this instrument was largely responsible for my recovery. I began to find that when people complimented me on my music, then all my fears and thoughts about food and my body melted away. In retrospect my eating problems and 'fear of food' were simply hiding my anxieties and insecurities around 'me' as a person. I always felt unworthy and perhaps to a large extent this was down to my parents. I can recall always being told that I was useless at everything (my mother still says as much, even today).

I also believe that, in addition, I am by nature obsessive–compulsive: I tend to become obsessive about things. For example, as a small child, I cried if models I made were not perfect. I possess an incredible amount of will-power, be it in my studies, diet or exercise. I think that I became 'high' on achieving things others couldn't.

Sometimes I wonder what would have happened if I hadn't exercised or dieted all those years ago, would I still have developed 'fear of food'? It is impossible to say, except that I believe that the dieting acted as a 'trigger' to a whole host of feelings and anxieties. Perhaps if I had drunk alcohol (I am teetotal) then that would have had a similar effect.

Losing my fear of food, in a way, was like losing part of me. I found a big void in my life that I have now managed to fill with other activities, but it was hard to give it up.

COMMENTARY – JIM BOLTON

Is someone a schizophrenic or do they have schizophrenia? Are they a diabetic or a person with diabetes? We try to make sense of a complex world by drawing conclusions based on limited information. As a result, we often describe someone as though they are their illness. It is as if we know all about them as a person just by knowing their diagnosis. A medical diagnosis does carry valuable information about what problems someone is likely to have and what treatment they need. However, the stereotype we attach to a particular illness is not only based on medical facts, but also on personal experiences and sometimes misunderstanding and fear.

What mental picture do you have when you think of someone with an eating disorder? You may know the symptoms that point to a diagnosis of either anorexia nervosa or bulimia nervosa, the two most common eating disorders. You will also be influenced by your own experiences. You may have had an eating disorder yourself, or have met someone with such an illness. You may also have gained information from the media, family, friends and colleagues. Our personal stereotypes are a mixture of all these ingredients, but there is a danger that some of our views are mistaken.

The attitudes and beliefs that lead to the stigmatisation of a mental illness are often based upon fear. Unlike many physical illnesses, mental illness can affect fundamental aspects of an individual's personality and behaviour. Sufferers may appear to behave irrationally and unpredictably. A natural response is to fear what we do not understand.

Symptoms from the two accounts of eating disorders include self-imposed starvation and vomiting, and obsessive exercise. All these could make them seem irrational. Through their behaviour they resisted the basic need to eat in order to stay alive.

What can be even more frightening about people with mental illness is that we might become like them. We have all looked in a mirror and wished we could change something about our appearance. Many of us diet to try and lose weight or exercise to improve our physique. If that wish to mould our bodies became all consuming would we become like them? We can protect ourselves from this fear by stereotyping people with eating disorders. It is more comforting to see them as so different from ourselves that we have nothing in common.

By stereotyping and stigmatising mental illness we strip someone of their individuality. A person with an eating disorder becomes an 'anorexic' or a 'bulimic', endowed with all our personal prejudices. These two accounts make it hard to hold such a view. Behind the starvation and vomiting and exercising is a person struggling to get out. There is someone with thoughts and feelings who might be like us.

The consequences of stigma

Our personal stereotypes of mental illness may have a basis in fact. Anorexia nervosa is more common in certain groups, including young Western women in the higher social classes. The author of 'Growing up' would fit into this group. However, there is a danger that such models blinker us to the possibility of eating disorders occurring in other cultures and social groups.

This difficulty in recognising an eating disorder that does not conform to expectations delayed her diagnosis of anorexia nervosa. She had to struggle against the wider views of society and her own attitudes and fears.

Gender

The author of 'Eating disorders in men' has shame about admitting to his illness was compounded by his gender. When groups of men and women with eating disorders are questioned there are differences between them, which are reflected in the two accounts. More often, men have been overweight and may have been teased or bullied for this at school. By contrast, women have more commonly been at a normal weight before their illness, but think they are overweight. Men will often focus on body shape rather than weight. Like the second author, they may pursue a masculine ideal of muscularity. Eating disorders in men are more common in groups in which athleticism and fitness are valued, such as army recruits and body-builders. However, at the heart of the eating disorders, the similarites between men and women are greater than the differences.

The heart of the illness

Both authors describe how their illness served an emotional role. For both of them the eating disorder became a protection against difficult feelings. He initally found a sense of achievement in the changes in his body, which reduced his feelings of inadequacy. Then a fear of regaining weight led to his rituals of exercising and starvation. More exercise in an attempt to build bigger muscles instead led to his body consuming itself for the energy it needed. However, the emotional pain in stopping was too great to bear and his weight continued to fall. She found that starvation brought an emotional numbness. It allowed her to resist growing up, bringing her physical and emotional development to a halt.

We all have to find ways of coping with difficult and painful feelings and to adapt to the changes that growing up brings. An eating disorder may seem to be the answer to this problem, but one that is physically dangerous and brings an emotional pain of its own. However, the way out sometimes appears more painful than living with anorexia or bulimia nervosa.

Conclusions

Personal experiences are an important way of tackling stigma. These two accounts of life with an eating disorder are made more effective by their emotional impact. We quickly lose the idea that eating disorders are all about starving and vomiting; at their heart they are more to do with difficult and painful feelings. The difference between an 'anorexic' and someone with anorexia nervosa is whether that person is their illness or has that illness. That is also something that these two people struggled with. Recovering from an eating disorder required them both to see their illness not as a part of them, but as something they wanted to be rid of. As these accounts vividly describe, that can be a long and painful fight.

COMMENTARY – MIKE HOBBS

More people than ever before are entering higher education, including significant numbers of people from backgrounds not traditionally associated with pursuing further education. These include students from socio-economically disadvantaged communities, ethnic minorities and from overseas developing countries; and people with physical and psychological disabilities who previously might not have managed independently in a competitive academic environment. There are students entering colleges and universities who are the first members of their family to pursue higher education.

Although higher education holds out the prospect of significant opportunity, it also involves a set of challenges that may highlight any vulnerability. Existing emotional difficulties and psychological disability may hinder the student's transition to independence and academic achievement, but the stresses of student life may also trigger the emergence of mental health problems for the first time. Although the student years are viewed as carefree and self-indulgent by many who have not experienced higher education, and indeed by some whose memories of college life are distorted by the rosy glow of retrospection, it is widely recognised that college students face significant challenges.

Students face a complex set of psychological challenges, for which their previous experiences of family, school and home life may have equipped them to a differing extent. Most students enter higher education in their late teens, and are still grappling with the psychological tasks of late adolescence. These include:

- progressive establishment of independence, both physical and emotional, which is particularly significant at the time of leaving the familiarity and structure of home and school. The ways in which students cope with this separation will be influenced by their previous attachment experience

- particular social pressures associated with transition from the relatively structured and prescriptive life of home and school to the permissive independence of college, including anxieties associated with establishing a new social network, making choices about interests and activities, and the perceived peer pressures to conform to new patterns of behaviour, including the use of alcohol and drugs

- bodily changes, around which there are particular challenges to do with sexual development, gender identity and bodily self-concept. A student may react to internal and external pressures by developing an eating disorder or one of its variants, including excessive physical exercise. The two accounts above give sensitive and insightful expression to the manner in which eating disorders may be manifest in students, and also how they can obstruct emotional, social and academic development

- contemporary pressures associated with (a) financial restrictions related to the present grant structure, the system for student loans and the increasingly common need for students to generate income to support their course fees; and (b) the competition for employment, particularly associated with increased expectations for material security and wealth.

The freedoms resulting from leaving home and school are associated with both challenges and risks. Self-confidence and self-esteem are key factors influencing a young person's decisions about the balance between conformity and independence. Psychiatric disorders, including eating disorders, may be maladaptive expressions of insecurity and the need for admiration, self-control and mastery.

Mature students may have the advantage of greater life experience than those who enter college straight from school, but may also face particular financial hardships, the added difficulties associated with supporting others (particularly children), and specific challenges to social integration. Mature students may feel less accomplished intellectually and physically too.

A different set of difficulties may be experienced by foreign students, especially those who are refugees from their own countries. Many foreign students will be struggling with adjustment to an unfamiliar language and culture, but refugees may also be suffering psychological reactions to traumas and losses experienced at home prior to escaping to the relative security of the host country. Fortunately, in most college communities the essential acceptance and humanitarianism of fellow students is much more likely to lead to empathic support and concerted efforts to integrate the refugee student.

The facilities in most universities and colleges for students with physical disabilities have improved in recent years, but they may face continuing limitations on access to certain institutions and courses; and physically disabled students must still deal with incomprehension and prejudice in some academic staff and student peers.

Much less progress has been made towards integrating students with problems of mental ill health. The potential stresses of higher education may not be adequately recognised by either the student with a psychiatric illness or the family and professional staff who support them, until a relapse is precipitated. Indeed, there has been a tendency to view higher education as a part of rehabilitation for students recovering from a mental illness. Although the opportunities for study and social integration may be fulfilling and productive, these students are likely to require sensitive support and continuity of their mental health care if they do relapse, and the associated interruption to or termination of studies is to be avoided. For students with existing mental health problems, the transition from home to college needs to be planned carefully, with active anticipatory liaison between home and college GPs and mental health services. Vacations, and interruptions to the programme of study resulting from further illness, require additional liaison as the student moves backwards and forwards between home and college.

For students who develop a mental illness after starting higher education, systems need to be in place for identifying emerging problems, providing support and counselling, and allowing the diagnosis and treatment of psychiatric illness.

Both accounts highlight some relevant themes. Insecurity in childhood may be associated with low self-esteem and lack of confidence; and, in the competitive environment of college, this may lead to a sense of inadequacy and unfavourable comparison of self with others. Second, underlying insecurities are heightened by the perceived loss of family, childhood friends and the familiar context of home and school, as well as the unfamiliarity of college life.

In addressing the mental health problems experienced by students in higher education, academic staff with pastoral responsibilities, college counsellors, GPs and mental health staff will need to recognise the developmental aspects of the students' problems. Mental illness in students can have a devastating impact on their academic careers if it is not managed sensitively and sympathetically. On the other hand, the developmental momentum evident particularly in young people can act synergistically with judicious professional intervention, leading to a rapid, dramatic and sometimes lasting recovery.

Eating disorders are illnesses that are generally believed to affect women, not men. However, with more men now contacting the Eating Disorders Association (EDA) than in the past, this has raised the question of what treatment and services are available for them. The EDA commissioned a review of specialist health care provision for men with eating disorders and published the results in February 2000 (EDA, 2000*a*).

COMMENTARY — STEVE BLOOMFIELD

The research aimed to gauge the incidence and prevalence of eating disorders among men in the UK, based on existing information, and to establish how specialist services provide for the needs of men with an eating disorder.

The EDA has long been concerned that investigation into the particular area of male eating disorder service provision has not been undertaken, principally because most people with an eating disorder are women. Nicky Bryant, former Chief Executive of the EDA, explains, 'As the instigators and publishers of the key documents on the purchase and provision of treatment services for eating disorders, we felt it was vital that a group representing about 10% of the population with an eating disorder should have their specific needs identified.' (EDA, 2000*b*) Although professionals are not surprised to see men with an eating disorder, they do need to respond appropriately and effectively to the differing needs and expectations of this group.

The overall findings identified a number of issues.

Incidence and prevalence:

- gender and sexuality are significant factors
- approximately 10% of people with an eating disorder are men, and approximately 20% of men with an eating disorder identify themselves as gay, twice the proportion of gay men in the population.

Accessing services:

- there are clear indications that the general lack of recognition of eating disorders makes it more difficult for men to access specialist services as their problems are less likely to be recognised and diagnosed by professionals, including GPs and psychiatrists
- cultural expectations make it harder for men to recognise in themselves that they have an eating disorder and need to seek help. For example, weight loss is more likely to be attributed to physical causes rather than to a psychological one.

Routes into the disorder

As there is less cultural endorsement for slimming among men, the onset of the eating disorder usually has a specific trigger, for example:

- avoiding childhood bullying or teasing for being overweight
- body-building or exercise
- specific occupations, including athletics, dance and horse racing
- concern of body shape and muscles in men (rather than body weight, as in women).

Men with a personal experience of an eating disorder were interviewed in the course of preparing the report and they raised a number of issues. The majority reported that their eating disorder had started in their school years when they were overweight and called names. Several reported being severely overweight in their younger years for reasons to do with low self-esteem and crises at home, and difficulties in coming to terms with the situation. For example, one man had been ten stone at ten years and was put on a 'diet' by the school. This led to him eating on his own and being teased.

The particular pressures in the gay male community to have the 'body beautiful' and 'be slim in order to get a partner' were mentioned by the four gay men interviewed. 'The scene can be a real meat market.' One of the men talked about the difficulties he had in coming to terms with his sexuality as a Christian and felt this had been a trigger for his eating disorder. The other gay men talked about the conflicts they had experienced when younger. It was felt to be a bigger problem in the gay male community than has been acknowledged, and among some men 'throwing up' as a weight control measure had become a normal way of life.

One man commented, 'Most men turn to alcohol and drugs as a method for coping but for some men an eating disorder is a way of coping with life stresses.' Four of the older men had experienced episodes of eating disorders throughout their lives, in relation to the loss of a partner, a relationship breakdown, a change of job, the stress of writing a PhD and so on.

Men also experienced particular difficulties discussing their illness with their peers. One young man commented, 'It is more difficult to come forward, you cannot admit to your feelings in a macho culture; people think you are weak and you fear that you are going to lose respect from your friends.'

The men were asked about their good and bad experiences of care and identified issues including easy access to sympathetic professionals who did not moralise but knew about eating disorders and could provide specialist help.

Some of the men had received a very prompt response from their GP; for example, it was a GP who identified that there was a problem with one of the young men when he saw him in town and referred him to a child psychiatrist. More commonly there was a lack of recognition by the GP of the problem or the severity of it, and this led to a delay in getting specialist help. GPs were seen as crucial, both because they often dealt with the men on an ongoing basis and because they had the power to make appropriate referrals and also to issue medical certificates. A number of the men reported that it was beneficial if the GP took a broader view of life issues, rather that just dealing with weight issues and doling out medication.

Two of the men had been involved with EDA self-help groups. Others had either not considered them, because they wanted to put the disorder behind them, did not know about groups in their area or were wary about them, for example thinking they might be the only man in the group.

The gay men highlighted the importance of having a visible gay male contact. One man reported that his partner had helped him a lot. Only one had experienced any service particularly aimed at men (the men's self-help group in Newcastle). He reported this as providing useful social support and reducing the isolation of the disorder. He now keeps in touch with another member of the group between sessions.

Reflections on caring

Philip Ingram

It started with my glasses. We were standing in the hallway, Pauline facing me with her back to the glass panelled street door. I forget why we were there, but everything else is firmly implanted in my memory. She stared at my face in a curious but strangely concentrated way. Then a smile spread across her own lovely features, and she pointed.

I couldn't make out what she was on about. Had I got a dirty mark on my face? I turned to look at myself in the hall mirror. No, the same somewhat dishevelled and perpetually worried expression stared back at me – no dirty mark or anything unusual.

By this time Pauline was convulsed with laughter. It was good to hear her laugh. Life, these days, did not often promote such spontaneous hilarity. Her Alzheimer's had changed so many things – for both of us.

'Look.' Her speech was already reduced mainly to single words and sometimes even these needed a room full of interpreters to understand. But the 'look' and the pointed finger actually touching my glasses now made it quite clear that it had something to do with my spectacles. I took them off, inspected them myself and then found Pauline looking deeply into my eyes. Years ago intimate eye to eye contact like that would have brought all sorts of notions into my mind that were best not pursued in narrow hallways. But these things had long since disappeared from our repertoire of togetherness.

We both examined the glasses still held lightly in my hand. Pauline touched them again but then lost interest. As I raised them to my face, I saw the door panel reflected in their curved surface, but, still none the wiser, I put them on again.

Then Pauline pointed at my glasses again and laughed once more. 'Peoples' she said. 'Little peoples.' Two words! Suddenly I understood. She could see her own silhouette framed by the doorway and miniaturised on the reflective surface of my glasses. I laughed with her and tried to explain what she was seeing.

I always tried to explain the things that Alzheimer's prevented her from sorting out for herself. We held many a one-sided conversation. I learned to construct short, simple, one topic sentences that Pauline seemed to understand – some of the time anyway. But I could never be quite sure.

Pauline, like most people in the early stages of dementia, was a great actor and was able to put on a performance of which any graduate from RADA would be proud. By acting the part of 'Pauline – a woman who had control of all her faculties', she had, so far, been able to hide from the casual observer most of the confusions that enveloped and tormented her.

The acting was obvious to me when the performance was directed at others, but it was more difficult to spot when we were alone. There was, in my mind, no need for her to pretend to me that she was more able than she actually was. I suspected, however, she had difficulties that even I, close as we were, didn't realise, let alone even begin to understand. The acting was for her own benefit – not mine.

Over the following days the reflections in my glasses stayed a source of amused fascination for her. We had many a giggle over them. We usually both tried to make light of the muddles in which Pauline increasingly found herself. Laughter is a great equaliser. Laughter healed the wound and the memory of it was soon forgotten – in Pauline's mind at least. Painful memories seemed to last longer with her.

The reflections in my glasses continued to amuse for only those initial few days. Slowly amusement changed to concern, the concern to worry, and then to fear. Sometimes this fear evolved into shear, unadulterated terror. If I came near her she became frightened, not of me but of those reflections. Her hand shot out and she tore the glasses from my face and hurled them across the room. This happened not just once but every time I went near her. I am lost without my glasses, but I quickly learned to remove them every time she got within grabbing distance. At least we were then both in the same blurred and confusing surroundings.

I thought of non-reflective lenses. Were there such things? The optician told me over the telephone that there were coatings that would reduce reflections. Come and see our samples. Not as easy as that. We lived in a village, a twenty-four mile round trip away from the optician and making arrangements for Pauline's care while I went took a few days to organise. I did eventually see the sample lenses but by this time Pauline's fear of reflections had transferred to other things. And life became more difficult – for both of us.

Mirrors caused panic, their surfaces and inner depths containing inexplicable terrors for her. I took them all down and stored them in the spare bedroom. I covered the mirror on the bathroom cabinet with paper. I stuck it down with masking tape that I planned to lift when I shaved. But as Pauline followed me everywhere, I was rarely in the bathroom alone, so I learned to shave 'blind' – less bother.

But all kinds of objects hold reflections.

Framed photographs and paintings behind glass had to be removed and stored. The spare room quickly became an Aladdin's cave of glitter and glass. The big picture windows generated huge reflected images and produced horror on a similar scale. So I put up net curtains to disguise. The glass doors on the display cabinets in the lounge had to be covered with paper. In the kitchen, the black glass doors on the eye-level ovens were similarly camouflaged.

Pauline saw reflections everywhere. The TV screen, the shiny plastic of the toaster and kettle held equal terrors for her. The light reflecting from the polished wood dining table caused apprehension. I caught her peering suspiciously at the far less shiny Formica surface of the kitchen table. It couldn't be trusted to stay that way. It was almost as though she found some masochistic pleasure in seeking out new reflective surfaces so that she could first get into a state about them, and then test my ingenuity in disguising the reflection in some way. Mercifully, for me, as reflections multiplied around the home, her interest in my glasses subsided. At least I could see what I was doing as I experimented by coating objects with Windolene, allowing the resulting chalky surface to dull any chance of it becoming another object of terror.

Strangely, there was one source of reflection that didn't trouble her, in fact it became a friend. This was the large square mirror screwed to the wall between two wardrobes and above a chest of drawers in the run of fitted furniture in her bedroom.

Pauline stood for hours in front of it talking to the person she saw reflected there. It was this person who became her friend. The friend was constant, always there, looked at Pauline, talked with her when Pauline talked, but had the decency to keep her mouth shut when Pauline wanted silence. She could share a good joke too. She laughed when Pauline laughed but when Pauline was sad and cried, she shed a tear as well. When Pauline wanted to sit quietly on the end of her bed, her friend kept vigil with her too. If Pauline became animated, her friend reflected the mood but when this turned to rage at what was happening to her, her friend instinctively understood and they ranted in unison. When Pauline wanted to get closer to whisper feminine confidences, her friend responded and also leant forward for the intimate exchange. They touched. They held out their hands to each other, fingertip against fingertip. I was forever wiping the evidence of these physical intimacies from the mirror's surface.

I should explain one apparent contradiction. Pauline could barely put two words together that made sense and yet she had these enormously long conversations with her friend. How was this? Fortunately her friend could understand what, to my undiscerning ear, appeared to be merely gobbledegook. But her friend not only understood it but also spoke it with great fluency. This was the mysterious language of those conversations. It was spoken with a full range of inflection, emotion and physical gesture. They stopped if I entered the room, so I often eavesdropped on the pair of them. The tone of voice and body language was quite explicit, but the words were in this foreign language known only to Pauline and her friend. Occasionally, just occasionally, the odd word of English was used as a source of emphasis, to make a point, or, perhaps, to fool an eavesdropper.

Caring at home

Gillian Harrison

How long? This question frequently crossed my mind after my husband and I began to care for my mother.

She had managed to stay in her own home in Birmingham for five years after my father died, but eventually her increasing dementia made this impossible. When she flooded her bathroom one night we brought her to stay with us in London, without considering the long-term implications. Nearly eight years later, she has just died aged ninety-two.

I am an only child and if we had known that the caring would go on for so long, the task might have seemed too daunting. Her repetitive questions and never having the house to ourselves all came as a shock.

Soon I had a desperate feeling of being trapped. As she could not be left alone overnight, impromptu get-aways became a thing of the past. Holidays had to be planned in conjunction with arrangements for her to be looked after. Suddenly we were even more restricted than when our children were small, particularly as my parents had always been willing babysitters.

To face caring long-term, it is certainly essential to keep life as 'normal' as possible. As I work from home as a freelance journalist, at least I did not have to give up my job.

At first we could leave her alone for an hour or two, though we took the precaution of having a safety tap put on the gas cooker. Later came disturbed nights (solved by a sleeping syrup) and wet beds (ditto by pads). Fortunately she never wandered out. Indeed, for the last three years she scarcely even tried to get out of her chair.

Our GP arranged for regular 'respite' stays in a special Alzheimer's unit – two weeks every three months. We could not have survived without them and my mother hardly knew the difference.

For several years she was sufficiently 'with it' to attend a centre run by Alzheimer's Concern Ealing at weekends – a change of scene for her and a break for us.

Initially she was at her most disturbed and disturbing in the evenings. Just when it was time to relax in front of the TV or read a newspaper, we got a constant barrage of 'Where am I?', 'Where are you, Gillian?' and 'I want to go home.'

No matter how close anybody was sitting and no matter how much we tried to talk to her, the droning repetition went on and on, impossible to ignore. But we were lucky that she expressed her frustration and anxiety only in words and never became violent, as some people with Alzheimer's do.

As her mental health declined, so the daily routine changed. At first, having been a very active person, she was constantly asking for something to do but could only manage simple tasks like peeling potatoes or washing-up. Though we have a dishwasher I used to leave a few dishes for her to do. Life became easier all round when she began to doze off more.

In her last year, when she could do nothing for herself, feeding took up the most time. Though she ate painfully slowly, she always enjoyed her food. Was this the only joy left in her life, I wondered? As conversation was virtually nil by this stage, I overcame the boredom by reading as I spooned it in.

People often asked if I found it distressing to see her getting more and more confused. Of course I hated losing my lively mother and no longer being able to have a sensible conversation with her. But you just have to get on with the task.

Seeing the funny side is important. One day I found her chatting to herself in a mirror. 'I don't know who that lady is but she won't stop talking to me,' she complained.

Naturally there were plenty of times when her slowness and stupidity were so irritating that I felt like hitting her (actually I only shouted). But even when she no longer really knew who we were, I believe she still sensed familiarity and love. Surely this must have been a comfort to her.

It is a great consolation to me that we were able to cope at home right to her peaceful end. Our three grown-up children were always willing sitters though I tried not to impinge on their social life too often as I would have hated them to regard their grandmother as a burden. In fact I think they would have been shocked had I ever suggested putting her in a home.

But the caring would have been impossible without my husband, who not only helped me but was prepared to look after her himself when I was away. In the last months he would often pop into her room to give her a Smartie. When he rattled the tube she opened her mouth. We knew her life was fading when she even lost interest in that.

I find it very difficult to write my thoughts on these two moving accounts of living with Alzheimer's disease. I have read and re-read them many times, and they

COMMENTARY – SUSSAN BENBOW

remind me of so many people whom I have met while working in old age psychiatry. Yet they're both unique and real.

I found it illuminating, but painful, to read Philip's vivid reflections on caring for his wife. He brings to life the reality of living with dementia. What it highlighted for me, as a doctor working with families affected by Alzheimer's, is the way that, as a professional, I can walk away, but as the husband of a woman suffering from Alzheimer's, he cannot. He is living with the dementia, just as she is. The dementia affects him as well as his wife: it is always there, through laughter as well as tears, touching every part of their lives. His account confronts me with the reasons why we try, in old age psychiatry services, to work with couples, families and friends rather than individuals. The illness doesn't affect individuals in isolation, and to try to treat them as 'islands' would be inappropriate: 'no man (or woman) is an island, entire of itself' (Devotions upon Emergent Occasions XVII, John Donne, 1571–1631).

In a different way Gillian makes the same point, as she describes how she and her husband, with support from their three adult children, coped with caring for her mother as her Alzheimer's progressed. The illness affected the whole family. They were all involved in it and had views on it. In some ways this makes the work of a professional trying to help the family more difficult, as the needs of different family members may conflict. As a professional I can join the family in their struggles to try to find the best ways of coping; different families will choose different ways and our job is to present the options and support their chosen route, which may or may not be the route that we ourselves would have chosen.

I salute Philip's inventiveness: the little things he did in order to try and help his wife make sense of her surroundings. These little things are the ones that make a difference, the things that professionals learn from carers, not from courses, books or lectures, but which we might be privileged enough to pass on to someone else in a similar situation. These too are the things that carers can share with one another when they get the opportunity at carers' meetings and support groups.

Another theme, which Gillian draws out, is that of the remaining joys or pleasures in life. She describes how her mother enjoyed eating when all else seemed to be gone. Philip's wife found an empathic companion in the mirror.

Gillian cared for her mother until she died and describes that as a great consolation to her. Some carers are unable to struggle on until the end, and their decision too must be supported and understood: just because their loved-one goes into care doesn't mean that the relationship is over or that caring has ceased, it just continues differently. Gillian's philosophy is 'you just have to get on with the task'. Some people can, but some people can't, and whatever their circumstances we have to try to help them through. They can still be the carer, even if their relative lives in a nursing home. They can still care, even when they can no longer bear to see what their loved one has become. Sometimes I think that not being there is harder than being there.

I can't write more. These pieces speak for themselves, and for the many people I've met in my work so far.

'Any man's death diminishes me, because I am involved in mankind; and therefore never seem to know for whom the bell tolls; it tolls for thee.'

Becoming ill

Jamie Barnes

My illness began in the summer of 1992. One particular day stands out in my memory. I had been to see an Andy Goldsworthy exhibition at Lancaster University with some friends. As we drove along the sea front afterwards, Steve put on a Jimi Hendrix tape at full volume. Nick saw my distress at the loud music and put his hand on my shoulder to console me. It didn't work. I reached over the back of the passenger seat and punched Steve hard in the back of the head shouting "TURN THE BLOODY MUSIC OFF; I HATE IT". He screamed out in response "THERE'S NO NEED TO HIT ME". Then I started a kind of intense sobbing and wailing. John stopped the car and we all went for a walk on the beach. The rest of the lads started messing about, drawing around each others' shadows in the sand and taking photos. The loud music became a big deal to me. I felt very emotionally sensitive, as if I were missing a few layers of skin. I was also suffering from mild psychosis.

Shortly after I spent a weekend at the WOMAD world music festival at Morecambe. I became taken over by everything in it; I talked to the musicians and stall holders, and even strangers in the street, about the music. I totally immersed myself in the experience. Although extremely hard-up at the time, I spent lots of money on weird and wonderful ethnic instruments and extra concerts. At the campsite I was in my element. I played the didgeridoo, the harmonica and the guitar, jamming into the night.

When the weekend was over, I began to form ideas about a new regime for teaching music; this preoccupation became an obsession, and subsequently a manifestation of the mania that I displayed in the first phase of my illness. I made copious notes and diagrams on a system of teaching that I believed could teach anybody how to play music. I distilled the playing of musical instruments into three categories: plucking, striking and blowing. Then I proposed simple rhythms to be played in a group, using my techniques. Next I recorded a tape of myself playing various instruments in rhythms that started off simply and became more intricate.

Around this time I had introduced myself to a local drumming teacher and music therapist. I talked to him at length on the phone and even hand-delivered a copy of the tape to his house very late at night. He confessed to me a few years later that he was very wary of me as he believed me to be a fanatic. He was right; I was on a mission.

A week later it was my university summer ball and The Pogues were headlining. I arrived wearing an old charity shop brown suit with a stripy Russian sailor's top and I carried an old cardboard suitcase containing dozens of copies of my tapes, a military bugle and a change of underwear. I also arrived with an agenda; to sell as many of my tapes as possible to raise money for the music therapist's charity. I even tried to get up on stage in the middle of The Pogues' set to spread the word about the charity. I was one zealous young man.

One night I was listening to the radio because I couldn't sleep. After about an hour it hit me. All of what I was hearing on the radio I was meant to hear; it was being said for me to hear; to help me. All the radio presenters knew my condition and were steering their conversations in such a way as to give me guidance.

Five hours later I was travelling on a train on my own, when reality came back with a great thud. Of course the radio didn't broadcast just for me, the presenters didn't know I existed. What I had experienced that night I can only describe as 'positive paranoia'. I believed everything was for me, not that everyone was after me, as in regular paranoia. Although dysfunctional, this delusory state must be similar to, say, a Buddhist monk who can only see the good in people. When the folly of this thinking hit me I began to cry – right there on the train, with all those people watching. All I could think was 'fuck, I'm ill'. It was then that I decided things had to change.

I saw a doctor the same day. I told him that I didn't know what was real anymore and that I knew I was ill and needed someone to understand me. I said I thought I was going insane. After all, I always was a touch histrionic. He told me that what I was experiencing at that moment was very common and it didn't mean that I was going insane. He said that I was, in medical terms 'hypomanic'; in plain English I was on the cusp of a nervous breakdown. Still on the cusp, mind. He told me I had the symptoms of extreme anxiety and unspecified psychosis. He said that the fact that I knew I was ill was a good sign. He prescribed me a few doses of temazepam: a tranquilliser that helps your mind to slow down and allows you to sleep. He told me to return in three days and he would think about dealing with the psychosis. He told me not to worry too much, 'I think we've caught this thing in time and we can nip it in the bud.'

Unfortunately, however, the doctor was wrong. It did get worse and two days later I was admitted under my own volition to the local psychiatric hospital.

ISSUES

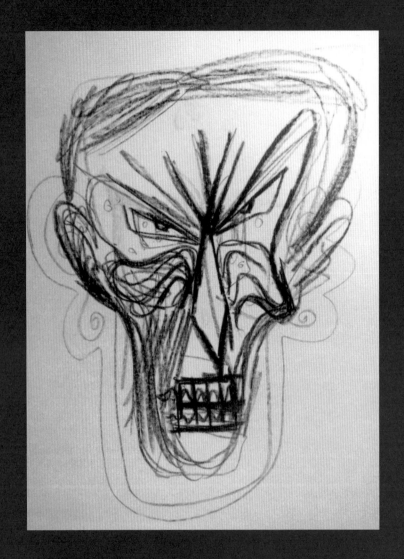

From the Adamson Collection

Suicide by starvation

Anna Paterson

Some cases of anorexia nervosa are linked to child abuse. This abuse can range from severe mental or physical torment, to bullying and neglect. Often this neglect or lack of love occurs in the first ten years of the person's life. The way people are treated in their formative years can have a profound effect on them well into adulthood. During these years our belief systems are formed and the way we view ourselves, our self-confidence and self-esteem are established. Anorexia nervosa is not about dieting. Weight loss is only a symptom of a much larger problem, which is why the media concept of anorexia as a 'slimmer's disease' inspired by thin models and actresses is so misleading.

From the age of three I was abused by my grandmother, who systematically tried to destroy me. Constant, cruel verbal taunts led me to believe that I was a bad person who didn't deserve anything good. I was a thin child but was never aware of this because she told me ,'You're a fat, ugly child and will grow into a fat, ugly adult.' As a child I was locked into dark bedrooms. I was offered presents, and then told I couldn't have them because I wasn't worthy enough. I was abandoned in shops for hours at a time.

My grandmother told me my parents would die if I spoke of the abuse, so I kept quiet. As I grew older and no longer believed my grandmother could kill my parents I still remained silent because I now felt I deserved the treatment I received. My grandmother's brainwashing was working. I felt I needed to be punished.

At the age of seventeen refusing to eat became the solution to my problems. The self-hatred was growing stronger each day. I hated my body, I hated myself and I felt I had to disappear. If I shrank in size then everything would be alright. To disappear I had to stop eating, which was fine because by now I didn't believe I even deserved food.

Like other people with anorexia I was being controlled by an inner voice that dictated my every move. This voice told me I couldn't eat, shouting loudly and persistently: 'You're a worthless, fat, ugly pig, disgusting, revolting and hateful. Stop eating now.' It was this all-powerful voice that kept me in a anorexic state, threatening that if I confided in anyone about my illness, I would be locked in a hospital and force fed until I was huge. Anorexia nervosa was my suicide by starvation. I was imprisoned in a nightmare world of terror, where food was the enemy.

I didn't consider that my own needs were important. I tried to look after everybody else and became especially protective of my parents. I shielded Mum from my grandmother. If I accepted the abuse then Gran had her victim

In anorexia nervosa, body weight is maintained at a minimum of fifteen per cent below the expected. Weight loss is self-induced by avoiding fattening foods and may be induced by restricting intake, exercise, vomiting or purging. There is a body image distortion evident as a dread of fatness. There is widespread endocrine disorder, which in girls shows itself as having no periods. Diagnosis for younger adolescents makes allowance for failure to gain weight at puberty and for delay in the process of puberty. Although not essential to make the diagnosis, social withdrawal, rigid self-control, obsessionality and perfectionism are common.

Within anorexia nervosa it is usually possible to identify difficulties in the areas of identity formation, independence, behavioural control and physical growth, which are the essence of the teenage years. Anorexia nervosa has the highest mortality of any adolescent disorder.

Most cases of anorexia nervosa occur in adolescents and young women, and, as the media often reports, it is linked to the extreme pressure on young women to conform to today's very thin role models of beauty. Underlying anorexia nervosa is often an adolescent maturational crisis, a combination of individual and family variables, leading almost inevitably to a crystallisation of the disorder. Research has found that serious negative life events occurred in the year before onset in a quarter of cases, but if such a life event had occurred this was more likely to be followed by a recovery.

Many children who go on to develop eating disorders in adolescence are free from neurotic traits and behavioural disturbance. They are often described as having been compliant, ideal children with a strong sense of morality, concern about the welfare of others and conscientiousness.

Chronicity is a marked feature of eating disorders. For the individual adolescent, weight loss usually increases concern with fatness, whereas increasing hunger usually increases the fear that loss of control may be catastrophic.

Anorexia nervosa arises out of a complex array of personal and family dynamics and, as Anna rightly says, it is vital to restore physical health to the young person but also that sustained physical healing remains a major treatment challenge.

Assessment and treatment of an adolescent with any disorder will only be effective if engagement in a therapeutic alliance can take place. The best way to ensure this is to understand not just the disorder, problem, difficulty or illness, but to understand from the perspective of the young person his or her unmet needs in all areas of his or her life. In turn this is enabling for him or her, hopefully allowing an adolescent to safely voice his or her inner pain.

In sharing her journey of abuse, pain, turmoil, hopelessness and the reality of anorexia nervosa, Anna shows us how important positive turning points can be in allowing us to form trusting, sustaining, relationships in adulthood.

If you prick us, do we not bleed?

Anonymous

One day, asking for a gay man's account of mental illness will be rather like asking for a Jewish or a red-headed man's. In other words, sexuality will be deemed irrelevant, unless sexual problems are central to the illness.

In my experience, that day is here, or should be. Depression, for instance, surely feels the same whether you're gay or straight. Other issues, in particular access to specialists and specialist services affecting all users, are far more pressing concerns.

I'm thirty-six years old. At the age of fourteen and again at nineteen, I suffered considerable anxiety and depression, and attempted suicide. I wound up in hospital both times, first in London and then Oxford. Similar problems, plus some bizarre somatising (sickness and dizziness in my own house), recommenced around the age of twenty-nine. Some of these problems continue to this day, though no more suicide attempts. I have been in psychological therapy of one sort or another for most of the past six years, both in San Francisco and London. I was on antidepressant medication from 1994 to 1996, and have been again from 1998 to today.

At fourteen I was told to attend weekly psychotherapy (no medication) at the London hospital I ended up in. The therapist was male. I have to admit that, over time, I notice that the gender of therapists seems to matter to me. I do better with men. Yet I've always preferred female GPs. The therapy worked fast – within three months or so we stopped meeting. Sexuality was glossed over; I don't remember it being mentioned. I already more or less knew I was gay and, perhaps unusually, was not particularly perturbed about it. I was, however, having problems adapting to a new, single-sex school, and maybe sexuality was an underlying issue. Perhaps it still is, but it doesn't feel like it.

At nineteen, in Oxford, I was discharged from hospital with the offer of psychological help, which I did not take up. (No medication.) As regards to sexuality, university life was liberal. By then I was openly gay, and all my friends (and my family, although it was not discussed) knew I was gay. In fact I very much enjoyed this openness. The depression, or whatever it was, was to do with acute fear (of what, I still don't really know), not sexual confusion. Over the years this fear/anxiety has been a persistent *basso continuo*. Interestingly, it presents itself virtually identically in my (heterosexual) father.

On arrival in the USA, things went wrong very fast. Within days I was extremely anxious, terrified. I felt I'd run to the edge of the world and had ended up hanging by my fingertips from a crumbling cliff-edge. My GP referred me to a psychiatrist. Access was almost instantaneous. Within a few days I was seeing him twice a week, fifty minutes per session. As I believe all psychiatrists do over there, he handled both psychotherapy and medication. The bizarre division in the NHS between hospital-based psychiatrists who recommend but cannot prescribe and GPs who prescribe did not exist. Meanwhile, I was at liberty to look for another clinical psychologist and/or psychiatrist if I wished to. At first, I did. It is common practice there to talk to a therapist at some length on the phone, or arrange a trial session, to see if you 'fit'. This rather astonishing choice was a little bewildering, but empowering too. There was no issue about catchment areas – they don't exist. There was no sense either that the service was short of cash, or that your treatment would be time-limited, or that you were in some way being weighed up for sufficient neediness, or that by receiving specialist help you might be preventing someone else on the waiting-list from being seen – quite simply because there is no waiting-list. The background guilt prompted by endless stories of NHS shortages is an issue for me and I'm sure for many other mentally ill people in the UK.

In San Francisco there were of course plenty of specialist units and individuals for treating gay people, including many openly gay professionals. I tested the waters but didn't like them. Like many gay men, I don't want to be ghettoised. I want treatment that makes sense in the real world, where I live, and whose standards match up to those of the real world too. Also like many gay men, I'm hypercritical of other gay men, vestigial homophobia perhaps. Moreover, I simply don't want to know anything about the private life of my health worker. Least of all his sex life. Of course, I wouldn't want to feel that my sexuality was disapproved of, but I have never felt this in either country, at least not from male professionals. I'm increasingly convinced that men are significantly different from women, but that gay men are not a lot different from straight ones. And the patient/professional relationship is a personal thing, the 'fit' depending on a host of issues, of which sexuality is way down the list.

In the USA things stabilised fairly quickly, medication being primordial in this initial stage. Various antidepressants were pretty expertly assayed then settled on and, in the first months, anxiolitics undoubtedly saved me from losing my job, which my boss had threatened if I didn't shape up in two weeks. Over time, the importance of this aspect of treatment declined; the psychotherapeutic side took over. I saw the psychiatrist for well over two years, initially twice weekly then once a week, fifty minutes per session.

I returned to England in good form. However, a year or so later, a fairly sudden crash caught the UK system on the hop, to say the least. My GP is kind and has a good reputation, but saw in me a problem that, she admitted, she felt insufficiently expert to cope with. To force me into specialist care she told me to present to casualty. Few experiences can be more appalling than a NHS hospital A&E department when you feel your world is falling to bits. For various reasons, among which a quite astonishing lack of empathy from the duty psychiatrists, this happened more than once. A period that I don't want to recall of bewildering attempts to gain real help from a system that seemed impenetrable or incomprehensible at worst, and random at best, ensued. Among other surprises, I was twice told by different doctors (once my GP, once a hospital doctor) that I needed help; the latter suggested three times a week, but that I would have to pay for it as resources simply weren't available. (Sitting on an NHS waiting-list to be told at the end of it that you need help that can't be provided by the NHS is distressing to say the least.) At one point I started seeing one of these private therapists: a clinical psychologist halfway across London who charged £80 per session. I believe he was gay, although this was, I think, a coincidence. I wasn't impressed and couldn't afford him anyway. After two or three visits I stopped seeing him.

A melée of other meetings around this time showed me that, in comparison with my previous US experience, funding, choice and access are not the only differences, although they are the crucial ones. Among the other differences, I'd highlight a much more conservative approach to medication in Britain, which may or may not be a good thing. There is also a surprising amount of labelling, of working in therapeutic 'boxes', here. Almost everyone I've seen announces that they're 'analytical', or 'behavioural', or 'cognitive behavioural', or whatever within the first few minutes; these schools start to sound almost like enemy camps. I rarely heard professionals define themselves like this in the USA. I would not suggest that one country is better than another because of this; I just make the observation. I would, however, remind professionals that the patient, at least initially, feels like someone in a burning building who does not particularly care what colour the fire engine is, or what depot it comes from, just as long as it puts the fire out.

My situation now is vastly improved. I could not possibly have written this a year ago, for instance (of course, among other things, I've learned that I'm going to have to take much of the responsibility for putting out my own fires, a message that is possibly more forcefully put in the UK than in the USA). I am comfortable with my progress, though not sanguine. I have to admit that in my current arrangements, I'm lucky enough to continue to see a highly experienced psychiatrist at a leading centre in London, once every six weeks or so for half an hour. This has not been entirely a matter of chance but also of contacts and pushiness on my part. He was recommended by a (gay) GP friend with more than usual interest in psychiatry. I personally contacted this psychiatrist. So it remains more than a little miraculous to me that his NHS schedule had room for me. In fact, given the peculiar way that he recommends medication but my GP has to write the prescription (a baroque oddity of the NHS's current funding routines, I understand), my GP knows I'm seeing him and has expressed mild, somewhat eyebrow-raised surprise that I have managed to be one of his patients. A helpful peculiarity of his practice is that it is not catchment-area specific. I believe this is very unusual. The normal reality – treatment by postcode – is tangible and stifling.

To wrap up the gay part. When suggesting this psychiatrist's name, my GP friend mentioned that not only did he hold him in very high regard, but that he was gay too, 'which can't hurt'. He's right, it can't hurt, but for reasons I hope I've explained, this information was pretty much irrelevant to me, and more than I needed to know. I have mentally more or less erased it.

Like heterosexuals, gay people with mental illness need access to expertise first and foremost. That has to be policy goal number one. The expertise needs to be truly expert, to be available to all, to be available fast and to be appropriate to the illness – not to the sexuality, race, waist measurement or hair colour of the patient.

Commentary – Michael King

This man's account of his experiences of mental health services addresses many issues. He has had treatment since adolescence for anxiety and depression, disorders that are common in his family. He understands how this must have some bearing on his own experiences but also feels daunted by his family history and worries if he will ever become well. He has managed to negotiate health systems in the UK and the USA and so holds an international perspective on what is possible and not possible, effective and not effective – for him. Our NHS does not come out of the comparison well, with confusing and slow referral systems, a rigid system of 'catchment areas', poor coordination of care and interminable waiting-lists. A&E departments pick up the pieces.

He is also gay, an issue that sometimes means people receive less than perfect mental health care. This does not seem to be the case for him. Nor has anyone, at least overtly, suggested that his problems arise from unresolved conflicts about his sexuality. We have little evidence over whether gay men and lesbians suffer any more mental health problems than other people because of societal and family prejudice. He is not particularly concerned about the sexuality of his doctor or therapist – that consideration came well down his list of priorities in determining who might be best equipped to help him.

The personal warmth and response of people from whom he sought help was of paramount importance to him. He was much less interested in their professional orientation or therapeutic stance. Being rescued was uppermost in his mind and I am struck by his impression that NHS staff sometimes seemed indifferent to his degree of distress. Do we become inured to the predicament of our patients as we see them daily? Does our response to their concerns become blunted by our routine? Encouraging our patients to write about their experiences of our services might help us to keep a wider and more sensitive perspective on their needs.

I'm a Somali refugee with seven children. I have been separated from my husband since I became ill in 1994. I have full refugee status and live in London. I'm unemployed. I've been in and out of psychiatric wards for the past five years. My present problem is as follows. Soon after my arrival in the UK things started. Whenever I try to go outside the house I always see two men with a video camera filming me and following in my footsteps.

For example, if I go shopping they are following me and waiting in front of the supermarket. Also there is a black man who works at the underground station who has committed serious crimes in the USA. He is also following me and wants to hurt me. At this time I was living in hostel accommodation, but when I moved to where I live now he also moved to where I moved.

He has fixed cameras at his house and films me whenever I come out of the house. Mrs Thatcher, the former Prime Minister, accuses me that I'm working for Sadam Hussein. Whenever I go outside the house I see two men with cameras, and their voices say to kill her and destroy her family.

When I applied for my flat, the council arranged an appointment for me. When I arrived at the council office I saw these two bags with video cameras inside them pointed at me, to film my movements.

Also, when I watch the television I hear the television referring to my name and my family name. I see on the television my hand and part of my body. The television is always talking about my children and says they will be destroyed and are refugees. They burn their country, they kill each other, why are they coming here to this country?

At the hospital I was asked to have blood tests and an X-ray. The X-ray department was fixed with cameras and computerised equipment and was filming my every movement. The staff were humiliating me and they beat me up and tried to assassinate me too. From that day I can no longer trust the hospital staff.

Refugees and mental health
SGH

The nurse told me that I have chest infection. Although I would like to accept the treatment I can't trust the hospital staff. I want to be treated for the disease because I don't want to pass it on to my children, but who can give me a guarantee that I would not be assassinated at the hospital by the people who hurt me before?

I was given a lot of psychiatric drugs but not to great effect.

The President of Russia also accused me that I was behind the Russian submarine in which more than one hundred men were killed.

I come from a family of two brothers and two sisters. My father was a nurse and had died. My mother brought me up with my two brothers and sister. In 1974 I got married to my first husband, who was an artist. I had little contact with him as he was not always with us. In 1988, when the war broke out in the north of Somalia (Somaliland), the people where I lived in Hargeisa fled to refugee camps in neighbouring Ethiopia. I heard that my brother was killed in the war. At this time I was living in the capital city of Mogadishu. I had a small business and was doing OK. I immediately fled to the north region to find my brother. After my arrival at the refugee camps I saw my dead brother and discovered that he was not dead, and his death was not true. Unfortunately, after I went back to the capital I heard that my brother and four of his children, two cousins and my mother were killed by meningitis, which killed many people at the refugee camps. Three months later the war started in the capital. Both the government and the opposition used heavy artillery and the city was destroyed within days. During this horrific experience I saw mass destruction and witnessed many of my neighbours hit by the artillery.

This time we had to escape from the scene and took a lorry to the north of Somalia. We had a very difficult journey as there were men with guns who were eager to take our belongings or even kill us. These men were shooting at our lorry and I was nearly hit by bullets on a number of times. When I got to the refugee camps in Ethiopia, life was difficult and we had to search for food and water the whole day.

We could not sleep in the night as there were flies biting us all over. We stayed there for almost seven months and then fled to Djibouti, where I stayed with a cousin. My cousin treated me badly and put me in the backyard of his house.

The climate was humid and I became weak and stressed. My husband was in England and sent me a visa. I arrived in England in 1994. I took two of my children to the school and the teachers did not welcome me at all and gave me unpleasant looks. At the school there were women taking pictures of me.

I was suffering from the trauma caused by the things that had been happening to my family in the war. When I went back on a visit to Somalia my problems disappeared.

COMMENTARY – DEREK SUMMERFIELD

SGH is unusual in two respects. First, she has been involved with mainstream psychiatry, including hospital admissions, for a number of years. The vast majority of asylum-seekers and refugees in counselling' settings are distressed but not psychologically disturbed (unless we are going to say that this is the same thing). Second, she now sees a Somali doctor in London. Although I do not doubt that the concerns recorded in this account have been authentically held by the client, it has been written up not by her, but by the doctor counsellor and (naturally) given a medical stamp. Doctors and patients do not always talk the same language: the patient brings illness whereas the doctor has been trained to make a diagnosis, not necessarily the same thing. This is, of course, no criticism of this or any other doctor, merely a reminder that a medical training tends to generate a particular way of seeing and organising what the patient brings.

To me as a psychiatrist this account does seem to lend itself to a diagnosis of paranoid psychosis and even schizophrenia – if I am to use an official (which means Western) psychiatric classification system. But psychiatry and psychology are Western cultural products, predicated on thoroughly Western ideas about human nature and the world, as well as on particular scientific and medical trajectories. Psychiatry makes universalist assumptions, made less resistable by the globalisation of Western culture generally, but what is its explanatory power in this case? Is a psychosis always a psychosis?

Although we must beware of characterising Somalis, or any other refugee population, as if they were socially, culturally and politically homogenous, we must honour the differences between this country and the Somali world. Their traditions, cosmology, expressions of distress and modes of help-seeking are generally different. So too are their definitions of madness (Somali refugees in Ethiopia use the term 'waalleh'), which is seen as capable of being caused by a physical illness, may arise for no known reason, or follow an extreme horror or shock ('argegah') or impotent rage and 'torn heart' ('marrora dilla').

SGH has persecutory concerns that seem highly personalised, wide-ranging, intrusive and persistent. What kind of disease is this? I note she dates this problem to her arrival in Britain, rather than before, and we will have to see if it recurs once she is back here. There are at least some indications here that psychiatry and its approaches have a less than firm grip in this case: is this because we are dealing with 'waalleh' rather than 'psychosis' or 'schizophrenia'? Her story certainly provides a basis for the 'argegah' or 'marrora dilla' that may precipitate 'waalleh', reflecting experiences of social turmoil, forced displacement, violent loss of loved ones as well as – no less influential – the shock of immersion in an alien city and culture.

In a foreign place, the sudden loss of familiar points of reference, the lack of language, the lack of basic knowledge and experience of how things work and of the nuances of everyday social encounters can lead to misinterpretation and undue suspiciousness. This may be reinforced, particularly in more vulnerable or distressed individuals, if staff in overloaded services are brusque. The promotion of negative stereotypes about asylum-seekers in the media and elsewhere contributes. SGH seems to be referring to the stigmatisation of asylum-seekers in one part of her remarks about television. Perhaps the teachers at her childrens' school were unwelcoming, perhaps they were not: either way, such perceptions are not uncommon among mentally well refugees. Nonetheless it is significant that her concerns have not waned with time and greater familiarity with life here.

COMMENTARY – KAM BHUI

Mental health services encourage users to play an active part in strategy, management and in some instances, service delivery. User satisfaction is one measure of the quality of a service. Mental health service users are being given a greater stake in the organisation and delivery of services, for example in consultations over the National Service Framework. Yet these developments will not automatically achieve a better service for users unless professionals share in the ambitions and vision of users.

Mental health service users from ethnic minority groups have specific dissatisfactions with services and professionals, as well as grievances about the overall quality of services received at a time when they are at their most vulnerable and in need. Ethnic minority mental health service users have to contend with prejudicial attitudes about their mental illness and their cultural origins. Institutionalised racism within health services and other public organisations compound these and contribute to a sense of powerlessness. The specific list of ethnic minority users' grievances includes greater risk of detention in hospital and less opportunity to use social and culturally acceptable treatment approaches, either instead of or alongside conventional treatments. Issues of choice and a perceived denial of choice further feed into the powerlessness experienced within mental health services. The reality for most ethnic minority users is that they come into contact with the very services they report to be insensitive to personal and private experiences of distress.

I believe it is the professionals who need to stimulate change in systems of care and how we conduct ourselves in our encounters with users and carers. We should remain fully responsible for the quality of care we offer, and we should be the driving force of change while being informed by and empathising with users' concerns. Professionals traditionally champion the services in which they work, always seeking to maximise the benefit to users of those services, but it has taken a great deal of protest from users for us to take their grievances seriously. We have to accept that we do not always see the obvious, and perhaps our roles and responsibilities, not to mention workloads, add to the level of insensitivity that we can show. Does user satisfaction really need to be a performance measure for change to take place? Do professionals really need a stigma campaign to prompt us to reflect on our practice? I would like to think not. However, we have these measures in place as a reflection of our inability to implement what I imagine we all wish to see realised within mental health services. Mental health professionals may be troubled by such challenges, as they are caught between the expectation that they are responsible for care if it goes wrong, as well as finding that the user movement is not sympathetic to the advice professionals give. Stigma is not only about mental health professionals questioning their attitudes, but this is one essential part of addressing stigma. My personal view is that as professionals we do not have the privilege of being wounded by challenge, but we do have the privilege of learning from challenges to our practice.

Falling through the net

Anonymous

I am a forty-year-old male. Just before my thirty-second birthday I was released from Wandsworth jail, where I served a six month sentence for deception. Upon release I was homeless, and St Martin-in-the-Fields' social care unit got me into a hostel for the homeless in central London in April 1993.

By the summer of that year I had got a good job, and I was drinking socially and smoking a small amount of cannabis. I was seeing the care worker from St Martin's regularly. I had a small shoplifting charge for which I got one year's probation so I was seeing a probation officer regularly as well.

I was going in and out of deep depressions, but still managing to hold down my job and save money while paying my own way at the hostel. I was the only resident out of some one hundred and twenty people paying their own rent.

I did not really have a social life in the normal sense. When I went out it was on my own, to pubs in the evenings, libraries, galleries and museums in the day. I was not taking any medication nor was I involved with any psychiatric services at this time. Life went on pretty much as it had done for the past five years, the pattern broken only by small prison sentences and bouts of heavy drinking.

In late summer I was interviewed and subsequently failed to get the room in the St Martin's home. I put this down to having a job and being able to pay my own way – soon after this I stopped going to work and started drinking heavily. I committed a series of burglaries for which I was never caught. I suddenly had more money than I knew what to do with, so began a two month bender. I was at this point very close to suicide. I realised I was out of control. After the bender, I went home for a long weekend at the end of summer.

The best way to describe how I was feeling now is probably disjointed. I had no cohesion in my life, seeing only the care worker from St Martin's and my probation officer. These were the two routines in my life. I did, however, get a place with Carr-Gomm Housing Association, but I felt out of place there surrounded by poverty and it got me down. I became depressed again and wished I was back in the hostel. I was also very angry and bitter about my life and situation. I had no ambition beyond finding enough money to drink and smoke cannabis.

The care worker at St Martin-in-the-Fields told me about a doctor at Great Chapel Street in Soho. I'd never been to a psychiatrist before and I did not know what to expect. I felt like a fraud because although I knew there was something wrong with me I could not see what the reason was myself. I told him about my depression and that I was breaking the law. I did not know what forensic psychiatrists were at this time. He gave me a prescription for some pills, which I gave away. I went to see him a few times after this but on one occasion it was someone different and on another occasion there were two doctors I did not know. I did not go back again and I never really talked the few times I did go.

I realised later on, while waiting to be sectioned for having a personality disorder and needing treatment, that had I been more forthcoming with the doctor at Great Chapel Street then this could have been avoided and there would not have been any incidents. But it was hard for me just to come in off the street and talk to a complete stranger about things I have been hiding all my life.

COMMENTARY – PHILIP TIMMS

The predicament described by this man is familiar – someone who has become homeless after leaving prison. However, he was able to make contact with St Martin in the Fields – a voluntary organisation that provides social services through a day centre in Trafalgar Square. With their help, he managed to re-establish himself in a job in spite of living in a hostel for homeless men and experiencing significant depression. This was no mean feat and demonstrates that he has substantial skills.

However, having a roof over his head was not enough. He was able to survive, but was not able to make new relationships. He felt that he needed a relatively high level of support and experienced troublesome feelings of depression. After his disappointment at being turned down for supported accommodation in a hostel, he returned to a life of crime and drinking. He had a brief contact with a psychiatrist and was eventually admitted to hospital against his will. Several themes emerge from his story – the vital role of voluntary sector agencies, the social isolation of homelessness, the difficulty in gauging the amount of support someone needs and the style of work needed to engage with someone who is socially marginalised or excluded.

He was effectively supported, not by statutory social services but by services provided by the voluntary sector. They gave help with housing and other practical issues and personal support. They enabled him to preserve a toehold in society but were, in the end, not enough for him to develop his inner resources. All too often, mainstream mental health services do not work closely with the voluntary sector.

Like many people, his outer capability disguised his inner fragility. His apparent self-sufficiency meant that he was not given a place at the St Martin's hostel and ended up in accommodation with much less support. He may have been able to cook, clean, pay his bills and even hold down a job, but could not tolerate being alone. He described himself as feeling 'disjointed' – a very personal expression of what it feels to be socially excluded. His only sustained relationships were with helpers – his St Martin's care worker and his probation officer. Consequently, hostel life seems to have provided him with a sense of belonging. This kind of experience has been ignored by much homelessness work, which has focused on moving people as quickly as possible to more independent and, potentially, more socially-isolated accommodation.

He did manage to see someone from mental health services, a psychiatrist, alone in a GP clinic. Whatever trust he had in the psychiatrist seems to have been compromised by the fact that on two occasions there were other people involved in the consultation. Whether these were doctors, students or nurses is not relevant. What comes through in his account is the sense of wanting a confiding relationship, yet finding this diluted and devalued by the apparently random appearance of strangers. As he comments, it was 'hard for me to talk to a complete stranger about things I have been hiding all my life'. This highlights the conflicting roles that psychiatrists may find themselves having to adopt. They include:

- the expert, who sees a patient, assesses him or her, pronounces a diagnosis and suggests a course of treatment, and then is no longer directly involved
- the teacher, whose prime interest is the education of junior doctors and other mental health professionals
- the 'personal physician', whose concern is the continuing welfare of the patient and whom a patient will grow to know and trust over a series of meetings.

Psychiatrists are specialists, so the roles of expert and teacher have been traditionally to the fore in their encounters with patients. However, with socially marginalised or excluded patients, this approach may not work so well. Diagnosis and treatment plans can be made, but they are unlikely to succeed if a trusting relationship has not been established. So, it may be that in this situation the role adopted by the psychiatrist has to be much more that of the personal physician rather than the expert or the teacher. The current shortage of psychiatrists in the UK means that psychiatrists are often put in a position where, because of lack of time, they have no option but to act as an expert. If this is the case, they must be able to call on other mental health colleagues who do have the time to continue and nurture the relationship. In this situation, multi-disciplinary work is not a luxury, but a necessity.

Ten years ago, when I was considering which speciality to follow, I worried about psychiatry for two reasons. One was the smoky environment on the wards and the second was the anti-religious sentiment.

The smoking has been dealt with; I no longer go home smelling like an ashtray. The second problem is still an issue that I grapple with. When I talked about becoming a psychiatrist my relatives feared I would be murdered and my friends feared for my immortal soul. 'Obviously' all psychiatrists are bitter atheists (with a beard and a Viennese accent).

During my psychiatric attachment as a medical student there was a distinct shortage of individuals willing to acknowledge a personal religious faith or even a spiritual dimension to existence. I was concerned that, as a Christian, I would be pushed to compromise my faith in my career.

In the UK, religion is often seen as a bolt on extra from the basic model, with Church of England as the default setting. In most societies, however, faith is at the centre of peoples' lives. Their religion gives meaning and structure to their experiences. To ignore religion is to ignore a fundamental part of many people's day to day existence.

Mental health professionals tend to be less religious than average and are often uncertain about how to respond to people's spiritual needs.

Doctors training in psychiatry are taught to consider the whole of a person's life: the biological, social and psychological aspects; the 'spiritual' is not normally included. In taking someone's psychiatric history we are told we must not avoid difficult areas, like their sex life and whether they have ever attempted suicide. Enquiry about their spiritual or philosophical beliefs is rarely mentioned.

Most of the major psychiatric textbooks touch on religion only as a direct correlate with race. This is an oversimplification because it excludes, for example, those who convert to a different religion and ignores the many variations within branches of the same faith.

There is a major overlap in the territory covered by a minister of religion and by a mental health professional. Issues of guilt and forgiveness, choice and responsibility arise frequently in both. However, psychiatrists are not priests nor vice versa. We must resist the tendency to expand the influence of mental health professionals outside their true sphere. Not all guilt is neurotic and not all low moods should be immediately medicated away. At the same time religious groups can be unhelpful, for example by pressurising their members to stop taking medication or blaming illness on lack of faith.

I did decide to train in psychiatry, the smoke fumes have dissipated and there has been growing interest in spiritual issues over the last few years.

A 'spirituality' special interest group of the Royal College of Psychiatrists was founded in 1999. This has provided a welcome forum for psychiatrists to discuss the area of mental health and religion and organise joint research.

Published in 1999, the Health Education Authority booklet *Promoting Mental Health* emphasises how Jewish and Christian communities can work with mental health services to support service users.

Specific journals (for example, *Mental Health, Religion and Culture*; first published in 1998) are growing in circulation. Research looking at the effects of religious faith on various physical and mental health indicators is increasing in quality and quantity (see, for example, the American National Institute for Healthcare research at http://www.nihr.org). There is an annual meeting on spirituality and mental health held at the Institute of Psychiatry in London.

In the future I would hope to see increased cooperation between religious leaders and psychiatrists to improve the recognition and treatment of mental illness in their particular community. In the West Midlands we are developing a project to educate church ministers in the early recognition of psychosis and clinical depression. The Avalon NHS Somerset Trust has led the way in linking chaplains directly with community mental health teams.

Mental health professionals need to recognise how their own views influence their expectations of what life is about and what is normal behaviour. Everyone has a world view even if they do not adhere to a formal religion. This world view influences our every action. If your culture teaches that all suffering is illusion to be accepted without struggle, then your behaviour is likely to be very different to that of someone whose culture teaches the need to strive to overcome personal weakness. All those working in mental health need ongoing training in cultural sensitivity, particularly for those who work in multicultural areas.

Religion and psychiatry have many areas in common. Increased understanding and tolerance on both sides will be to the advantage of all.

Razor sharp roses and cartoon clouds
Race through the sky and burst from the ground
Chimneys seek heaven, the fox hunts the sound
Of life unseen beneath our eyes all around.
Badger he yawns in his sett down the hill
Harold the heron sharpens his bill
Margaret and Ivor with a view to a kill
A glint of fish all dressed in gold
Dressed up for dinner, tickets all sold.
Magpies crackle so coarse and so rude
Indignant that they have as yet got no food
Mice with a half life of a mouse if in luck
Spend their lives with a dive and a duck
For a morsel, a crumb, a seed in some muck
All outside my back window.

If my mind was my own would you leave me alone?

The Lighthouse man

My great grandfather
Was a lighthouse man
Two weeks off
And four weeks on,
He cooked his dinner
At half past one
And he always
Had fish on a Friday.

LIVING WITH…

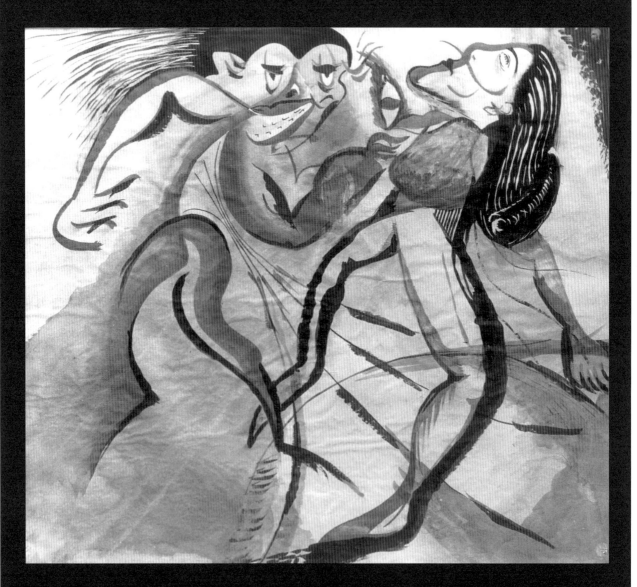

From the Adamson Collection

My in-patient career

Anonymous

This is a section from a longer script. It is about one long in-patient admission. It is mainly about the role of ECT in the treatment of acute depression.

In 1990 I was a part-time senior trainee in psychiatry and mother of three children aged two and under. My history of affective disorder extends back to the age of twelve.

I had been ill for much of the preceding year, from mid-pregnancy, responding to an antidepressant but relapsing within weeks of the birth. Therapeutic contact did not get to grips with my illness before it overwhelmed me months later prior to my psychiatrist's temporary desertion on annual leave. A brief 'respite' admission was arranged. It lasted for almost six months.

Leaving my children with my mother on admission was distressing and I shall always remember the care of a young student nurse at the beginning of his first placement. Later I remember supper, put on the floor outside my door: all white – mashed potato, boiled white fish, washed out grey-green courgettes exuding a pool of liquid into the white sauce. I ate nothing.

As I no longer had to do anything for other people, there was no need to do anything for myself. So I stopped – speaking, eating, drinking. It is difficult to describe what it feels like to be depressed to that degree. Suffice to say there is an absence of feeling, a lack of engagement with the world, rather than acute pain or suffering. I didn't really miss my children while in hospital.

Presumably because of my profession, I was deemed to have capacity to consent to ECT. Like all junior psychiatrists, I had administered ECT earlier in my training and so was acquainted with the procedure. I always knew it would happen to me some day. I signed the form.

Deeply withdrawn and passive as I was, the atmosphere was one of inevitability. I was not particularly afraid or anxious and no coercion at any time was required. The ECT suite was unusual, with an oddly shaped windowless anteroom, grey, dim and cold. It had a strange, amateur painting on one wall of a path leading past a squat palm tree to a closed gate in a high wall. There were no figures in the picture. After too long a wait the reassuringly friendly, cheerful figure of the out-patient nurse emerged to summon me. The chamber was much more technical looking than the place I knew from work, mostly because of banks of anaesthetic equipment. I cannot see it, be there or think of it without simultaneously thinking 'lethal injection'. Various associations come to mind – euthanasia, punishment, passivity, defeat, release, peace at the last. Particularly peace at the last. (I have never actively sought to end my life.) I lay there unresistingly while it was done to me – oximeter on the finger, the needle, anaesthetic rising cool up the vein in my arm, knowingly submitting…

Memories did not register again until I was back on my own bed and I had no significant side-effects – perhaps the occasional headache. Longer term, my memory was reversibly affected in textbook style, particularly for names during the following few months, most embarrassingly when my dual worlds of patient and psychiatrist first coincided, but it was of no real consequence.

I had a series of eight treatments, with substantial improvement, then started going home on leave and relapsed comprehensively. Another series of eight treatments followed before I was discharged to the day hospital, which I attended for several more months.

Of course ECT wasn't the only treatment I had. There was medication too. Antidepressants in quantity, plus for some weeks mid-admission a large amount of a major tranquilliser as I was agitated. This was something of which I was not subjectively aware. Even when outwardly retarded, thoughts can be racing internally without a means of expression. I can appreciate that the psychological also wasn't neglected.

Ward life was enclosed, almost a ritual – an orderly sequence of days and occupational therapy sessions. I would sit on the terrace (behind high reinforced perspex screens) staring over London into nothing during those muggy August evenings. Later I got up in the winter darkness to await the morning shift and the first cup of tea in the empty smokers' lounge to breakfast TV. I don't recall many visitors.

I have had two more series of ECT treatment since then. More recently recurrences of my illness have been managed pharmacologically. There are pros and cons. Personally my choice would have been for more ECT because it is quick and I know it works for me, but because I am now recognised to have a bipolar disorder it may be prudent not to use a treatment that theoretically could push me from depression to hypomania (though it did not previously). I am still seeking stability.

Jake's hospital journal

Jamie Barnes

The hospital was an enormous Gothic cathedral of a place. On the walls of the corridors were painted flying angels, some with trumpets, others with harps. I saw a doctor who asked me what was going through my mind. I went into a long, disjointed and gabbled diatribe about my subject of the moment: science and art.

After my parents and Andre had left, I was called back in to see the doctor. He started asking me questions and then a weird thing happened. I began speaking 'in tongues'. What I mean is that I started answering his questions in different accents and funny voices. I have no explanation for this whatsoever. While he was talking to me a beeper on his table kept going off every twenty seconds or so. I was convinced that this meant he was hypnotising me to extract the true answers from me.

After the interview was over I was sitting on a side-ward by myself staring at the wall. There and then I experienced a hallucination. I saw the form of a trumpet on the wall. It went round in a square loop and the bottom of the trumpet then turned into a map of Australia. I thought that this meant I should travel to Australia to find myself.

When my sister came to visit me at the hospital, I had become completely preoccupied with my left and right and which should be black and which white. I had a white packet of cigarettes in my left hand and a black lighter in my right hand, and I was trying to work out in which hand each object should be.

Then a strange and frightening thing happened. I felt a great pain in my back, as if someone was cranking up my spine. My head stretched backwards and I was bent right back until the nurses gave me an injection that slowly made my muscles relax. I still don't know whether the great pain I felt was due to my condition or a side-effect of the medication.

The obsession with left, right, black and white continued. As I walked along I had to chant 'Black, white, red. Black, white, red…' Black was left, white right and red the centre of my head. I also took to wearing sunglasses because my eyes had become very sensitive to light. In the queue at the hospital shop a bloke asked me why I was in hospital. I replied that I was afraid of the colour red. He was shocked and said how sorry he was. Every time someone asked me this question I gave a different answer. My fears had such a high turnover; my mind was spinning so fast.

The ward was okay; it was like a bizarre holiday camp, with free drugs. The rest of the patients were fine mostly. We had quite a good laugh sometimes; getting up to mischief, playing music, drinking lots of tea and smoking lots of fags. At one point I was even under the delusion that the patients were all actors and had been picked for their similarity to people I knew to make me feel comfortable. I also thought that everyone with dark hair and dark eyes, like my own, was directly related to me. I believed that the whole world was made up of three or four enormous families.

I became quite good mates with a man who believed he was a reincarnation of the tragic folk singer Nick Drake. I think this guy had schizophrenia. He used to sing Nick Drake songs loudly in the common room and he even changed his name to incorporate that of his alter-ego. Another patient thought his parents were robots as he could see metal beneath their skin. Apparently this bloke was a high-powered lawyer. Nick thought he was

but for the staff who may not be adequately trained or have the time to work on these areas. The Sainsbury Centre for Mental Health suggests that 'insufficient attention to social needs identified by patients…could be perpetuating the revolving door pattern'.

One of the most common complaints that service users on the wards bring to us is that staff do not spend enough time with them. There are pockets of staff who do not work in a respectful way with service users: making time to talk, listen to and support people during difficult times. This input is greatly appreciated by service users when it happens.

There is, however, a commonly held view that staff are often too busy to be able to sit and talk. It can seem that staff spend a lot of time in the nurses office dealing with crises, completing necessary paper work or just having a chat.

The number of agency staff on wards is a financial concern to trusts but more importantly is a service quality issue in that the use of agency staff who may only be on a ward for one shift during a person's time in hospital does not allow for trusting relationships to develop.

Access to one's consultant via the weekly ward round can at best be an opportunity to discuss one's concerns and negotiate changes to the care plan. Ward rounds can also be an intimidating and unfriendly process that leave people feeling frustrated and out of control.

There can be a reluctance to share information with individuals about diagnosis, medication, side-effects and care plans. This lack of sharing is sometimes caused by poor communication systems on the ward and at other times seems to be based on a professional's perception that it is 'better' that the person concerned doesn't know.

The sources of the inadequacies listed above are multifaceted. Adequate resources must be in place to ensure that basic amenities and trained staff are available to all users on acute and intensive care wards. Staff training must emphasise individual experiences of mental distress and focus on ensuring that people are treated with respect and dignity.

But perhaps the first step is to clarify the role of in-patient care. Are wards simply custodial holding places for people or are they meant to provide a safe and therapeutic environment for people in distress?

The adult I may have become

Sarah Swainston

I sometimes wonder who I would have been if I had not become mentally ill. At seventeen I was head girl at school, doing well in my A-level course and on target for entry to medical school. From eighteen to twenty I was a medical student, doing reasonably well and enjoying life. At the age of twenty-one, I suddenly and unexpectedly crashed into a depression that lasted several months and required ECT even to begin to lift it. At twenty-two I returned to medical school better, but a different person. Once you have looked into that black empty hole, the memories never quite fade.

But I was young, on the whole optimistic and assumed that my life would continue on its previously smooth road. I knew that I had lost contact with some of my friends but it never occurred to me that I might have lost contact in a way with my previous self.

Over twenty years later and following several more episodes, it has finally dawned on me that I have never grieved for that lost twenty-one-year-old. It was brought home to me by a film *Shine*, which is about a brilliant young pianist whose future is suddenly shattered by a devastating psychiatric illness. I found myself crying for him – for whom he could have been, what he could have done, the relationships he missed – and I thought, 'what about me?' I've been much luckier. I've got a family, a career and a husband. But, I still wonder – how would I have been different if I had never been ill?

When someone loses a leg we understand the loss; when a couple has a disabled child, we recognise that they need time to grieve for the other child they never had. When working with an adolescent with a chronic illness we try and help them come to terms with the fact that they may never have a future. But when working with a young person with mental illness, do

COMMENTARY – WINSTON McCARTNEY

I have often heard people say that good comes from suffering and strength from adversity. Having mental illness myself and working with fellow sufferers on a daily basis, I see little evidence of any truth in such maxims. I suspect Sarah would agree. I think for many who live with mental illness the plight of the mythical Prometheus is sadly typical. Prometheus stole fire from the gods, and for this he was chained to the rocks where an eagle ate at his liver afresh each new day, so his suffering continued. Only the efforts of Hercules could break Prometheus' chains and free him. I like this story because the fire we have come to possess, those attributes that set us a little lower than the gods – our intellectual capacity and our creativity – can also bind any of us in the chains of madness that for some can mean a life of unrelenting suffering. As Sarah points out, once you have looked into that black empty hole and can see no way back out of the darkness the memories never quite fade. The individual's personality may be changed.

People often assume that depression has a clear aetiology with an insidious onset. This is not the case and Sarah's almost instantaneous decline into depression, which appeared to come out of the blue, is not untypical. John Stewart Mill stated:

'Over himself, over his body and mind, the individual is sovereign.'

For those with depression, loss of dignity and self-respect often ensue, as does the loss of personal identity. Sarah mentions the loss of contact with her previous self and the loss of the adult she may have become; those with depression often have little sovereignty over their own mind and body.

I have never thought of depression as a grieving process. Anger, denial and acceptance are not part of most psychiatrists' lexicon when helping someone cope with depression, yet it makes so much sense. Depression changes your relationships with those around you, changes your social activity and the pattern of your working life. No wonder then that Sarah experienced anger and may even have engaged in scape-goating, looking to those around her as precipitators of her illness and the cause of new bouts of depression. Others look for theoretical constructs, (helpfully) provided by eminent psychiatrists such as Freud and Laing to justify this blame game. Perhaps more than most, those who suffer from depression tend to be insular and introspective, constantly looking for meaning in and reason for their suffering. The truth is, sometimes none are to be found and the onset of the illness transcends any psychosocial construct.

Sarah's long period of denial and failure to accept her illness is so common. The problem is compounded by the stigma of having and admitting to a mental illness (even psychiatrists are not immune to stigma) and, of course, the widely held belief that an illness like depression is not a real illness like cancer or coronary heart disease and, therefore, could not be as debilitating. People often feel fraudulent and that they have to 'get on with it'. Those with mental illness don't get much of a sympathy vote and so Sarah, in carrying on with such a demanding career, put in place all the factors that would ensure the recurrence of her illness. Those of us who live with depression always want to beat the illness, always want to overcome it and regain the previous self. The vast majority of people who have a bout of depression can regain their former self, but for some people like Sarah and me, the hard lesson is that we cannot beat the odds and we must come to terms with the need for change in our life in order to treat and manage what may be potentially a lifelong illness.

So to sadness and acceptance. Sarah tells us that she will let us know if she ever accepts her limitations. I you ever think of it in terms of the loss of the adult they could have become?

There are, of course, stages of grief; when I was much younger I was angry with everyone who, however unjustly, I felt had made me depressed. When I am depressed I wish I could apologise for the hurt I caused during that time. When I am well I know that it was understandable and I really have nothing to feel guilty about.

The next twenty years were spent in denial. I would never admit that I could not do everything I wanted to and blundered on, occasionally falling off cliffs – getting patched up and on my way again. Again I was lucky. I had family and friends who tried to support me and would have done more if I had allowed them. It must have been extremely hard for them at times, watching me carrying on as though nothing had happened. I was also lucky in that I had colleagues at work who stood in for me during the times I spent in hospital and supported me on my return. It was particularly hard, working full-time and studying for exams at the same time. It has always seemed as though the number of things I am doing at once has been a major factor in the recurrences of my illness.

So what about sadness and acceptance. I do feel sad for that young student from the past and I'll let you know if I ever accept my limitations. However, I'm gradually learning a difficult lesson. When I had my first child I decided to work part-time. Luckily this coincided with my first consultant post and I did not have to go through the procedure of becoming a part-time trainee. Although this worked well for a while, I found that that job was not particularly suited to part-time working and the stress began to build up. Eventually I moved to another part-time post, but following several months of severe depression and two hospital admissions, I decided to retire from the NHS. I now work privately, concentrating mainly on medico-legal work. I enjoy this as I can control my own workload and above all have time to think about what I am doing. I even have the luxury of time to study. I miss the NHS, the friendships, the teamwork and dedication. I could not cope with the relentless pressure of waiting-lists. It is a limitation I finally have to accept.

I have also, I think, accepted that I cannot pursue as many interests as I would like. I have a number of hobbies, but if they take up too much time, they become a stress in themselves.

I know some of the ways in which depression changed my life. I would never have become a psychiatrist for one. I had my sights fixed on plastic or trauma surgery, until I learnt that I could not cope with the long hours and disrupted sleep. I would also have had a more settled and stable personal life during my twenties. On the other hand I might not have met my husband and had the children I have now. I would not wish to change that.

think she already has and her career to date shows that she has taken personal responsibility in her working and personal life to ensure that the risk of recurring depression is minimised. It is terribly sad that the misunderstandings associated with mental illness, the trauma and dramatic long-term psychological and physical effects that depression can have, are so little appreciated. This is why it takes so long for many of us to accept our limitations. Without wishing to minimise anyone's suffering, it may be easier to accept the debilitating effects of heart disease or kidney failure.

Now back to suffering, adversity and good. Sarah's sadness in not being able to achieve what she wished to do will be shared by many and although there would seem to be no Hercules to unbind Prometheus, perhaps there is good among suffering. For Sarah, her successful family and professional life, and for all of us, the fact that she became a psychiatrist. I know that her remarks will resonate with many others and I hope that her fellow health professionals learn from her experience and apply it to their patients.

Living with severe mental illness

Paul Reet

I suffered a period of severe depression for nearly four years. I was the head teacher of a village primary school and the stress of the job, along with other life events, forced me into my depression.

I did not know what was happening to me and I felt physically and emotionally drained. I became anxious about the slightest of things, with surges of emotion rushing through me, leading me to feel dizzy and tired. I was not sleeping and I lost nearly five stone in weight. Work became an obsession to the exclusion of everything else in my life. I could never seem to get on top of anything and I remember feeling like a rabbit trying to get out of a hole and being pushed back in all the time.

After much persuasion I saw my GP, who referred me to the community mental health team. My community psychiatric nurse (CPN) advised me to take antidepressant medication. I was on this for over three years but it never relieved my symptoms for a sustainable period. I began seeing the CPN once a week. He used cognitive therapy to challenge me about my distorted thinking related to my feelings and coping strategies. After two months he referred me to a psychiatrist who explained that I had experienced 'burnout' and needed to rest, eat and exercise.

Despite taking up all the advice I was offered, things began to deteriorate and I was finally admitted to the local psychiatric hospital. Although this time away from home helped to relieve the stress on Mary, my wife, I did not receive much help from nursing staff on how to deal with my distress in the institutional setting. I clashed with my named nurse on more than one occasion as I was growing frustrated that she could not make me better. My cognitive functions were affected and some of the nursing staff did not appear to understand what I was going through. The one person who did help me at this time was the physiotherapist, who, following on from the advice of my CPN, encouraged me to work out my stress through physical activity and at other times just walked with me in the hospital grounds, talking and listening.

The symptoms of my distress ranged from feeling very angry and frustrated, crying, sleep walking, pulling my hair out, thumping pillows and a feeling of wanting to run away all the time. When I was at home my distress got so bad that I cut myself with knives and felt a great sense of relief from hurting myself. In the end Mary had to hide any sharp instruments in the house.

My third admission to hospital was in March 1996 and it was decided that I would have ECT treatment. After the first two doses I began to feel that the pressure was lifting; suddenly the sky was bluer.

When I left hospital I continued to see my CPN. He also referred me to a psychologist, who systematically worked through with me the life events that had contributed to my illness. These included childhood experiences, my work obsessions, our infertility problems and two tragic deaths.

All through this time Mary and I had the support of my CPN, who was always there for us and always consistent with me. He never put me under pressure but had a way of helping me face up to my feelings and distorted thinking patterns. He slowly built within me strategies for coping with stress that I still use today.

I began doing some voluntary work for a homeless charity after I was finally retired from teaching at the age of thirty-five. By February 1998 I had stopped seeing the CPN.

Within a month I began hearing voices and I was admitted to the hospital following a visit from the psychiatrist at home. He took me off all my drugs, confirming to me that my symptoms were not depressive in nature. I did not understand what was happening to me and I got so desperate that I tried to take my own life at least three times. Eventually my distress eased without medication and I was able to face up to a personal issue for which I sought private counselling.

Since this time I have become actively involved in service user issues to improve provision and understanding of mental health services. My wife and I regularly talk to nursing students about our experiences as a carer and user, respectively.

In September 1999 I started my mental health nurse training with the intention of making a difference in service provision and care for mental health sufferers. I am a Christian and believe that what has happened to me was for a purpose. I remember writing in my diary back in 1995 when I was first ill that although I could not understand what was happening to me I knew there was a greater purpose behind all this. This has been proven to be true.

COMMENTARY — ROGER FREEMAN

This man has clearly had a serious illness – he had become a head teacher in his early thirties and had to give up his profession – he lost 'nearly five stone' in weight and later needed ECT. Now he has made a good recovery and is training in a new profession, which happens to be mental health nursing. His illness was a complex one that, from his account, does not follow a usual pattern of illness. I suspect that his professional carers found him difficult to assess and to treat.

Paul's account of his illness is full and thorough. It begins sounding as though he is one of those people I have regularly met, who are often teachers, who find that the stress of the different, and usually extra, achievements expected of them in their work in the past ten years or so is too much. The stresses, together with a biological vulnerability to depressive illness, lead to serious symptoms, like Paul's anxiety and weight loss, for which, like many men (rather than women), he did not seek professional help until much too late. I wonder how he got to his GP. Was it his wife who eventually persuaded him, or was he pushed by his employer or work colleagues because he was obviously unwell? Did he have a formal psychiatric interview with a consultant psychiatrist? I hope so. He does not mention it, but that does not mean it did not happen. Sometimes overbusy community mental health teams protect their members by not referring on clients they are getting nowhere with, as this generates yet more work. He should have had a full investigation of his physical state (given, particularly, his weight loss) and also a thorough discussion of relevant life events both with him and, with his consent, with his wife, right at the beginning. He himself only mentions life events later, after his third hospital admission. He says these were systematically worked through with a psychologist, but a few months later he went for private counselling with 'a personal issue', rather than back to the psychologist or another team member, which I would have expected if a good therapeutic relationship had been built up.

It is a shame that there was such a clash when Paul was in hospital, between him and his named nurse. Paul puts it down to his frustration at not getting better. Paul might now like to consider, with the wisdom of hindsight and his new experience as a nursing trainee, that this frustration may have been a feeling that the named nurse shared. It might have been better if it had come out into the open. I do not know what to make of the hallucinations episode, and am less convinced than Paul that his symptoms were not depressive.

I am glad that Paul has found a new career – but surprised that he was accepted for mental health nurse training so soon after having had both symptoms and considerable treatment. I hope that he gave his illness history to the occupational health doctor before he started the training. It was appropriate to take him on for training, but special arrangements should be made for him to have some support easily on request if he feels he needs it; and, in the interest of his patients' care, for a senior member of the training staff, with his consent, to be made aware that he had had problems in the past. Then, if any further difficulties arise during his training they will be picked up and help can be offered as quickly as possible. Sadly, his commitment to Christianity does not ensure that there will not be any difficulties, although firm beliefs can help contain people's personal difficulties.

Controlling cravings

Anonymous

I started 'using' alcohol twenty years ago when I was seventeen. My drinking grew steadily worse until my life became so out of control that I was at risk of losing everything – job, home and even life itself.

I was admitted to hospital for detox and stayed for six weeks. At first I was so relieved to be rid of the physical agony that I suffered every day in withdrawal. I felt quite positive and thought I had been 'cured'.

After leaving hospital, reality hit me. I felt depressed. I suffered terrible mood swings. Sleeping was very difficult. I began to feel 'hard done by'; I was sober so why didn't I feel better? I began to wonder if it was all worth it. How could I carry on without my bottle of self-esteem, confidence and comfort? I craved for drink constantly.

My problem was that I was not used to feeling my feelings because for so many years I had used alcohol as an anaesthetic for them. It became clear to me that in order to continue in my recovery I had to learn how to bear these feelings – face up to them, own them. I found this daunting, the pain and anger were often unbearable, but I knew that drinking again was not the answer and that it would only result in more agony. I couldn't live with alcohol or without it.

This state of ambivalence continued for nine months. Then I took a drink again. I can't say that I was being complacent because deep down I had a sense of impending doom – I chose to ignore it.

Within less than one week I became physically hooked again – suffering shakes and sweats and nightmares but this time it was worse, the fear that I felt was immense and added to that was the overwhelming sense of failure. I was so angry with myself that I didn't want to carry on. I felt very suicidal.

Eventually I was admitted to hospital again and had another detox. This time it was much more difficult – I had almost given up hope.

Somehow I managed to pick myself up again with the help, support and encouragement of the staff, my friends and family. I was so grateful and realised I could not conquer my problems alone. With their help I rediscovered my inner strength and the will to go on.

During my time in rehab, I started to learn how to connect cravings for drink to feelings. They were more familiar to me and were mostly of anger, sometimes sadness, loneliness, fear, jealousy, guilt. Often I felt as if all these feelings were combined. I described this as the 'black hole' – an endless cavernous emptiness in the pit of my stomach, which was so overwhelming that I felt I would die from it.

Well, I didn't die from it – I learned to live with it and before long it became less powerful. I did not allow myself to make the connection between feeling bad and wanting a drink, I would simply acknowledge the feeling and feel it. It was also very tempting to fantasize about drink – these fantasies were of pleasant, sociable drinking where the situation was well controlled. When I found myself slipping off into this imaginary state I would quickly remind myself of the first night I spent in detox and the agony I went through. I would also force myself to remember awful situations that I had been in while drunk. This was, after all, reality for me.

Using this method I began to feel better; it was such a relief not to crave for a drink. It dawned on me that feelings were not always awful ones anyway and I noticed that although the bad feelings were more painful, the good feelings were more pleasurable.

Today I feel well physically. I am also beginning to reap the benefits of living in sobriety; in control of my life, I now get things done more efficiently. I wake up in the morning without a sense of shame or despair and I can remember everything that happened the day before. Also, for the first time ever in my life, I have a little money saved.

I know that this is how I want to continue my life. It's not always easy staying sober, but as time goes on it does become easier. I feel confident now but I am very aware of how easily I could slip back to rock bottom again.

The difference is that instead of just existing from one drink to the next, today I am really living my life.

COMMENTARY – ROGER FARMER

This account illustrates vividly many aspects of alcohol dependence. The author started using alcohol when he was seventeen, and the seeds of dependence are often planted in adolescence. Recreational, occasional drinking may lead to a pattern of more regular, excessive drinking. In some occupational or social circles drinking is acceptable or expected. Some people find that drinking helps to dampen down anxiety or despondency.

Certain factors may make people more likely to become dependent on alcohol. There is evidence that certain types of personality or mental illness, or a person's genetic make-up may increase the chance of this happening. However, if anyone drinks enough alcohol, frequently enough, for long enough, that person will become dependent – no one is immune.

Eventually, because of the response of the body's nervous system to alcohol, withdrawal symptoms are experienced if a person does not continue to drink alcohol regularly. The author mentions the 'physical agony' he suffered every day in withdrawal. These physical problems include shaking, excessive sweating and feelings of sickness. In more severe cases people drink in the mornings or even intermittently during the night to top up the amount of alcohol in their body to try and prevent or reduce the withdrawal symptoms. Another aspect of the nervous system's response to continued heavy drinking is called tolerance. This refers to a person's need to drink more to experience the same effects.

In this account the writer described sleeping being very difficult even after leaving hospital. Insomnia is common for weeks or months after withdrawal. Alcohol, in common with certain other drugs such as benzodiazepines, can affect both the amount and the quality of a person's sleep. When someone stops drinking there may be an increase in 'dream sleep', causing nightmares and insomnia.

He also describes the problem of rapidly re-developing dependence (in his instance within one week) when someone drinks again after a period of abstinence. This may be due to irreversible changes that have occurred within the nervous system or to psychological conditioning.

When someone becomes dependent on alcohol his or her drinking habit is likely to become predominant, to the detriment of family, friends, work and so on. As a result people may lose many of these supports, so rebuilding a life without alcohol is more difficult and a person may need help with rehabilitation in a hostel or day programme. This man was lucky to have support from his friends and family after his second detoxification programme. There is evidence that having such support, or having a job, makes recovery from alcohol problems more likely.

Although withdrawing from alcohol is an important first step in recovery, in the longer-term there may be many psychological and social difficulties a person needs to face. These may include quite profound lifestyle and even spiritual changes if someone is going to replace using alcohol with more beneficial habits. It may be almost like going through a bereavement, with feelings of loss and grief for that familiar but self-destructive relationship with alcohol. People may find it difficult to be alone and face their feelings without the buffer of alcohol. Everything now seems more direct and immediate. Pleasurable feelings are more intense but so too are painful ones and these may be difficult to bear. Perhaps also during the years of heavy drinking people have avoided negative experiences and feelings so they have not learnt how to tolerate or cope with them. The author describes clearly the painful feelings that he confronted when trying to stay abstinent. Gradual awareness and acknowledgment of both positive and negative feelings allows them to be less overwhelming so that a person can feel more in control.

After withdrawal from alcohol there continue to be strong desires or cravings for alcohol even many months into abstinence. These desires may be sparked by feelings, as in this case, or by certain situations such as passing a bar or meeting a previous drinking companion, although sometimes they seem to occur out of the blue. Over time, if a person stays abstinent they usually become less powerful, but this information can be of little consolation when in the grip of intense cravings. Distraction, for instance by contacting a non-drinking friend perhaps through Alcoholics Anonymous, may be vital.

People need to be vigilant in avoiding or coping with situations that might involve drinking for many months and often years into abstinence. This account underlines the importance of forgiving oneself and coming to terms with the past, as feelings of shame are common. Generally people develop the resolve to overcome alcohol problems and change their lives when the disadvantages of continued drinking outweigh any benefits. In rebuilding one's life, this time without alcohol, positive, happier and more fulfilling alternatives to alcohol will help to keep the balance tipped towards abstinence.

Under a cloud

Barry Lane

Where on earth do I start? I am an ordinary fifty-year-old man with a wife and grown-up children. Through a lifetime of tranquillisers I have plunged to the depths of wishing to end my life, never able to go out far, never able to walk into a café, never able to eat out, in fact never able to live a life. After struggling through the years I am now normal, even able to holiday abroad.

Why do I need to write this account? Apart from my wife Sandra, I never had anyone to talk to. How lovely it would have been to confide in others.

It all started way back I suppose. Nerve problems led to the first prescriptions. When on a holiday in the Lake District, we wanted to go on a boat trip. We walked around for what seemed like hours waiting for me to pluck up courage, then I took a tranquilliser and waited for it to have an effect. Eventually we went on the trip, but of course I felt ill and never enjoyed myself. I tried to hide it as much as I could, but while away had to seek help from a doctor. His words were, 'Why have you come on holiday when you are as ill as this?' He gave me a different tranquilliser. Life was a struggle.

As a family we used to go to speedway meetings at the local track, but I suffered before, during and after the meetings. Waiting for the racing to start I would feel ill. When it got underway my mind was taken off the pills and I could at least enjoy some of what was going on. After the meeting, my wife and the two girls liked to go to the pits and meet the riders. I always wanted to get home, so we would leave early. What a way to treat your family. Years later I still have this terrible guilt at how I deprived them.

I also loved football and many times I was asked by my workmates to go and watch Norwich City play. Time after time I would turn their offers down. Little did they know how it scared me. Year after year when watching my local side I would huddle under the trees, all alone, continually looking at my watch and wishing the game away so that I could go home. Beforehand, I would have taken another dreaded tranquilliser, hoping it would make me feel better.

I think that, to my credit, during this time I never used my troubles as an excuse to take time off work. My doctor thought that it might be a good idea to take a break from work, but

I always felt that I had to continue. My workplace was two hundred yards from home but then, to my horror, the firm was to move twenty-five miles away. What was I to do? I still had to support my wife and two girls. The firm moved so I went with them. Worse was to come when my mates started taking their lunch at the pub or the local café. Going out to lunch was too difficult. If only I could turn back the clock and show my former mates how I now love going into the pub and that eating out has become a pleasure.

One day I arrived at work to realise that I had forgotten to take my pill before leaving. Sandra had to drive over to me to deliver it. Then the firm I worked for went bust and closed down. I was out of work for the first time in my life at the age of forty-three. This was nearly the straw that broke the camel's back. I did get a nine-week temporary job, but I was getting worse. In October 1990 I was offered a job by an old work mate. The work was very exacting, quite complicated and began to push my limits. I managed to cope.

This is where the long road back started. The job changes, meeting new people and new situations had eventually tipped me over the top. I needed help. At the first appointment with the therapist I sat and talked and talked. He told me I had to learn to relax. With the aid of an audiotape I had to go through a set of exercises every night after work. Night after night I had a hot bath, lay on the bathroom floor or on my bed and went through a routine of relaxing each muscle in my body in turn. Hoping and praying for the miracle to happen. It never did. I was getting no better.

I went back to my very understanding GP in the depths of despair. I think he realised that I might even be contemplating suicide. He suggested I should go for specialist help. This turned out to be the turning point in my life. With Sandra by my side, we went into this wonderful man's office. There was no 'pull yourself together' or 'snap out of it', but the promise that he could help me. I poured out my troubles in tears. A box of tissues was handed to me and words of encouragement that I was ill. Just very ill. Not going daft. He was going to wean me off the addictive tranquillisers and replace then with a non-addictive drug.

The next session of the treatment was hard to endure – coming off the tranquillisers – 'cold turkey'. I was at the same time introduced to the new drug and warned that it might take many months to get me better. I went through many terrible side-effects. One of them eventually stopped me taking baths because when I was in the water any small movement seemed to make the water rock and shake. Another was of terrible bouts of perspiration, sometimes even waking in bed in a pool of sweat.

My doctor was marvellous to me through this terrible time. Constant visits to him reassured me that all would eventually come good. The dreaded tranquilliser doses were cut down and down. I was nearing the day in my life that I was never to forget. I stood at work in my usual daze when all of a sudden it seemed as if a miracle had happened, a cloud just seemed to lift from me. I suddenly felt normal.

I would sit and talk with my father-in-law about all my problems. Little did we know at the time that he was much more in need of help than me as he was slowly dying from cancer. In the past I would have been a jibbering wreck, but because of my improvement I was able to help console Sandra, the girls and my mother-in-law.

A year after Sandra's dad died, my mum passed away. I coped admirably. My mum left just £300 to me. This money, I decided, was to help Sandra and me, especially me, try and achieve a tremendous goal. I would add to my mum's money and this would enable us to make an excursion abroad.

The trip went brilliantly, which did the world of good for my confidence. Suddenly all the impossible situations from my past were being conquered. Then my mother-in-law was taken ill and within a fortnight had died from cancer. Our three remaining parents had passed away in the past three years. We coped.

Now Sandra and I go off on our own, making up for all that lost time. So you see if you are suffering as I was, there is light at the end of the tunnel. I am no longer afraid to tell others of my former problems, but perhaps it is easier now that I am better.

Getting better

Janet Powick

I understood my schizophrenia extremely well as I received extensive psychoanalysis in the 1970s, by an analyst I met by chance. Because of this, one night I experienced a 'waking dream', in which all the pieces of the jigsaw fitted magically into place. I had the answer, the cure and now all would be well. This, however, was not the case. I developed a schizophrenic reaction that seemed to erase this dream from memory. It reappeared slowly over a period of years.

I met Barry, my present husband, ten years ago. He is an uncomplicated man, with no hang-ups that I am aware of. I told him about my mental illness on the first date – initially, subconsciously, I must have thought he would not bother again. His reaction was, 'So what!' I was flabbergasted, because it was definitely not the type of reaction I had experienced previously. It was more understandable when he told me that his first wife had been epileptic.

The relationship continued into engagement but, although I loved him, there was an underlying anxiety that I could not dispel. The anxiety got worse, and I asked him if he was trying to take over my personality. The feeling was of an extremely physical and deeply psychological nature, causing my own person to become extinguished. His reply was, 'No chick, I am not.' This was an overpowering memory from the past. The adult part of me knew it was not true, however, the child in me could not let go. I slipped into schizophrenia; it was the worst episode I had experienced. Barry cared for me with genuine compassion, and I felt comfortable with him.

In the daytime, while he was at work, I had to go to my mother's house as I felt I did not exist without her. If I existed within her, somehow I would still be alive. The anxiety was so acute, I learned to float past it with the aid of a book I had read on how to control nervous suffering. I floated when I was in a panic in queues in shops and so forth. I could not do anything practical, so Barry did all the cooking on the previous evenings. He encouraged me to stay in bed in the mornings, something I was never allowed to do before. The first time this happened, it was snowing outside and Barry said, 'You are in the best place, darling.' I stayed there all day, until I was fed up. After I arose, I felt motivated, simply because I was allowed to do something that had previously been forbidden.

Barry bought me a puppy, he was so cute and I felt comforted by stroking him. It helped to pass time and drive away the most unbelievable thoughts. I had to realise that the destructive voices I heard were not real, but part of a delusion. When I had these thoughts, and the paranoia, Barry would sit down with me and encourage me to go back like with the psychoanalysis, to find out where they came from. When we discovered the source, the thoughts started to disappear. Although I was still depressed, I was thinking a lot more coherently. I was only just discovering that it was OK to talk about my illness. Back in the 1960s, when it began, there was so much shame and stigma, that I was heavily discouraged from discussing it with anyone. When I appeared in front of psychiatrists, I was unable to tell them the truth. Hence my diagnosis did not appear until I was thirty-seven years old. The particular breakdown at the time was so intense that my GP noticed the schizophrenia in my face.

The habit of visiting my parents' house in the daytime continued until Barry suggested, 'Why don't you try not going today?' I panicked, how could I exist without my mother? I would be alone except for the puppy. It might be alright; after all, a puppy is alive isn't it? I remained at home all day, stroking the puppy. I remembered something Freddie (my analyst) talked about in psychoanalysis. The fact that there was an invisible umbilical cord attached between me and my mother, and that I would have to cut it in order to become a separate emotional human being.

When I was a small child, a voice told me that eventually I would become an artist. Teachers encouraged my talent at school. I became prolific at painting and won several competitions. However, whenever I had a schizophrenic episode creativity stopped until recovery, when I experienced an ultimate creative explosion.

Since my recovery, Barry has supported me through university. I was awarded a first class degree with honours in 1997 for sculpture with printmaking from the University of Wolverhampton. In my final year I was encouraged to make work that highlights the plight of the mentally ill. The next year I won a bursary from the British Academy in London to study full-time for an MA in fine art, which I was awarded in 1999.

Sometimes, according to certain events, I can experience thought disorder and paranoia. Freddie would have said, 'What does it remind you of?' Barry and I work as a team dismantling events, finding explanations within my experience, until there is nothing left but thin air.

I owe my life to Alfred Frankl (my analyst), who died in 1992, and my husband Barry.

Being a gay carer

Mark Paige

'Oh hello,' said Peter's chiropodist, 'You must be his son.' 'No,' I said, encouraging her to have another go. A look of embarrassment passed over her face. 'Oh no,' she said, 'I'm sorry, you're his brother, aren't you?' 'No,' I said again, 'but keep on working at it, you're sure to get there eventually.'

She smiled and three toenails later you could see the truth starting to dawn on her. Desperate to be seen to be sympathetic and desperately trying not to ask any further questions, she completed her work and thanked us both and moved on to her next client.

'There we go again,' I thought, 'another coming out unavoidable and reasonably successfully achieved, but not without the usual cost to my own feelings.'

That is how it's been during the past five years. Seemingly endless people in far too many situations, who should have known better, seeking, sometimes demanding, reasons why I, a man, am caring for another man. And each time it happens it becomes necessary to produce the same stern eye contact as I silently dare any of them to produce any response other than acceptance, once I have explained. If I receive empathy then it is a bonus, though I have tended to get that from my gay friends. I have come to the conclusion that in the short-term if only we had gay hospitals, gay residential homes, gay whatever, where you don't have to go through this threatening process, it would make this carer a happier one. Some time ago some gay friends placed a relative of theirs in the same home that Peter is in and the feeling of solidarity during that brief period was very valuable for me.

I tell myself when I feel insecure that the experience of needing to come out is necessary for the sake of those in the same situation, who will come after us, and to an extent that is true, someone has to lead the way. But for me there has been more to it than that because the coming out is only the start; active acceptance also needs to follow. All too frequently these days you get merely 'PC' acceptance, which avoids judgement, meets the letter of equal opportunities, but fails to signal any sort of warm welcome. Even people I work with in the local Alzheimer's Society branch enthusiastically receive my contribution to their activities, but very few ask me how Peter is; that would be taking things too far.

So, for me, it has become necessary to force the issue on all comers, though it has never been at the expense of Peter's dignity. At the residential home, where he now lives, I realise that I am making a conscious effort to show that the quality of my caring as a gay man is as good, if not better than that of other carers. When he kisses me, and he does tend to do that rather frequently and in any situation too, then I receive it as any partner might. When there are social occasions organised by the home I always try to be there and will treat my presence as normal as that of all of the other carers. At our carers' support group I ensure that my experiences are delivered with as much weight and matter-of-factness as any of the others given, so that the added issue of sexuality cannot arise. And when there is a cause for celebration, such as his birthday, it has sometimes been held in the residential home rather than our own home, if only to make the point that we belong there too. Some of my gay friends have dealt with these issues by calling their loved one their 'brother' or their 'business partner'. I came to the conclusion a long time back that loving care for my own loved one could only be delivered if I loved myself with honesty and integrity, and if that meant doing so with an in-your-face approach, then so be it.

In the world of dementia one is invariably surrounded by elderly people whose lifestyles and experiences inevitably reflect a different world. They are usually married, and those marriages have often lasted many decades; they are also likely to have families surrounding them too. My relationship carries decades with it too, but it also brings with it a lot of baggage, which is distinctively gay, valued and which I do not wish to discard simply because my partner has been placed in a non-gay environment. I value the years of laughter we have had and this continues even though it stems from Peter's behaviour. We laughed when he called our priest 'Father Christmas'. When he started stealing things and brought a whole roast chicken home. When we moved him to a better room in the home and he continued to sleep in the original one, even though there was also a new female in it (good for his image). When we try to get him to do the actions to 'YMCA' and he gets them hopelessly wrong. The laughter is always followed by hugs; the behaviour of the rest of us is no less irrational at times.

Our relationship carried with it no agreement to be faithful to each other and I now have a lover who is as concerned and understanding about Peter as anyone I could have wished for. Some non-gay carers have been horrified by this fact, but this new experience, and the others I have referred to, are signs that as more gay people succumb to this terrible disease, caring for them will not be a matter of slotting them into already existing schemes, but will demand fundamental changes in understanding, approach and activity if some of the worst experiences I have received are to be avoided.

Commentary – Jill Siddle

In this commentary I have tried to identify some common elements and link them to my own experiences as a carer of two sons with mental health problems.

At first sight, these narratives illustrate three very different people coping with completely different types of illness. Yet a number of similarities also emerge. As well as areas of concern, there are examples of good practice, which hopefully will be of help to others involved with mental health issues.

In each case the narrator has had to overcome considerable stigma and distress before a positive outcome could be achieved. My own experience as a carer extends over a long period as my eldest son, now in his mid-thirties, had his first serious clinical depression when he was fifteen. Although there have been many bad times, again there is a positive outcome as good family relationships have been maintained, he is married, in full employment, has appropriate professional support and his illness is well-managed.

What are the key elements that bring about improvements? In the case of my eldest son, and in Janet's and Barry's accounts, that describe the length of time it took to find appropriate help, the turning point seems to have been the intervention of a knowledgeable and caring professional who eventually provided the correct diagnosis and treatment. Why, in these different situations, did it take so long?

One common strand seems to be that some doctors were continuing the same treatments for many years without questioning the diagnoses; they were not having a true dialogue with the patients and families to try and develop their understanding, acceptance and management of the illness. Only in recent years does it seem that the majority of doctors have realised that they should explain illnesses and treatments, both to patients and carers, and involve patients in taking responsibility for their own health.

Another factor is that, as a by-product of the ignorance and fear surrounding mental illness, many patients are frightened to tell anyone about their symptoms and so delay asking for medical help, or feel unable to ask for a second opinion. In the accounts relating to schizophrenia and tranquillisers, many years of suffering could have been avoided if there had been an understanding in society that most mental health problems are due to an illness and that successful treatment is available. Patients and their carers could then have sought help without feeling shame and guilt and learnt to accept that these problems were not in some way their own fault.

Having received the correct diagnosis and treatment, what else do these success stories have in common? In every case there has been loving and consistent acceptance, support and care from those in a close personal relationship with the patient, such as a partner or member of the family. So how can we ensure that both essential professional and personal support is available? It took many years and a number of painful hospital admissions, with constant changes of psychiatrist and opinion, before my eldest son, and the rest of the family, could accept that he had a serious illness and needed regular medication to keep well.

Five years ago my youngest son also became mentally ill, at the age of twenty-three, and in his final year at university. It is only in the past year that he has been helped to come to terms with his illness and accepted that he too must take responsibility for the necessary limitations to his lifestyle and the disciplines of daily medication. If only those who think of mentally ill people as weak could see the courage, perseverance and determination needed by patients who cope with these disorders, often with inconsistent and inadequate professional support, as described in the varied experiences described here.

One aspect that is not dealt with in these accounts is the anguish of many of those caring for someone with a mental illness, particularly in the early stages before self-management is achieved or at times of crises, which can be extremely traumatic. This is often exacerbated by the general lack of information, understanding and support provided for carers. It would be interesting to hear the views and feelings of the other family members involved. No one would consider the needs of all mental health patients to be the same, yet carers are often placed under one umbrella. Although at times most experience the anxiety and pain of seeing a loved one suffer, the problems and needs of those caring for a partner, parent, sibling or child are very different, even if the carers are grouped according to the diagnosis of the patient. Without the necessary support, caring for a parent or family member over many years can prove insurmountable for some with a resulting breakdown of the relationship.

If the correct help is provided, positive outcomes are possible for those who live with the consequences of mental disorders. These personal stories, together with my own experiences, demonstrate that the stigma, stress and strain often associated with mental illness can be overcome. With timely diagnosis, appropriate treatment and care for patients, on-going and sympathetic support for carers, there is a strong likelihood of finding light at the end of the tunnel.

Growing up as a carer

Nicola Dacre

I am fifteen years old. I first met my dad when he started seeing my mum when I was seven. He later married my mum when I was ten. No one knew then that he had Alzheimer's. He had a poor memory but everyone thought it was the stress of his job. He was fifty-three.

It was hard for me because he would tell me to do one thing one day and then the next day he would say I was wrong. I thought my new stepfather was rather strange.

It was hard for my mum too because she would ask my dad to do things, like paying bills or making phone calls, and he wouldn't. Then they would argue.

When I was eleven my dad was told to give up his job because as an orthodontist he could have given the wrong treatment to someone.

I didn't hear the word Alzheimer's until I was about thirteen, but I had heard words like senile dementia and CJD as possible causes.

He changed from being nice but forgetful to someone who shouted at me. Sometimes I hate him even though I help to look after him. All my mum's attention goes to him and not to me.

When he goes in for respite care my mum and I can do things together, but it isn't very often.

Now my dad is much worse. He wanders off and goes to the toilet in his trousers. He doesn't always know who I am even though I help him.

My mum and I are much closer now because we look after him together. I wish he would get better. I never had a dad and I would like one now but I wish he didn't have Alzheimer's.

My mum works but looking after my dad is very hard and she gets ill a lot. She doesn't want him to go into a home and neither do I but one day I think he will have to because we won't be able to manage.

We now have a carer who comes in and baths and dresses my dad and makes his breakfast before he goes to the day centre.

I don't like being alone with my dad because he doesn't like me trying to help him and so he shouts at me.

Every other Saturday I go to the Young Carers Connection Group. It is nice to meet other young carers and some of them are much worse off than me.

I used to have trouble with my schoolwork but counselling has helped. Sometimes, if it is difficult at home in the evening, I don't work so well the next day. The school didn't understand at first but my mum told them what it is like to live with Alzheimer's and now it is better.

The Young Carers project came to my school to talk in assembly. My friends didn't really understand, but they are supportive. Some make fun of me.

I wish my mum didn't work so hard and I wish I had a proper family. I've never had one.

When my dad was getting worse no-one talked to me about it. They said I wouldn't understand but I did know what was happening and I would have understood if they had tried to explain.

Everyone asked how my dad was but no one ever asked how I was. It was three years before anyone realised how much it was affecting me.

It became increasingly difficult to care for my dad at home.

One day in July 1998 he went to the day centre and never came home again as he had become violent and it was considered dangerous to have him at home. He was admitted to an assessment ward and then later to a long-stay ward. I had mixed feelings about this at the time, as I was relieved he was not coming home but sad that this had become necessary.

My mum and I visited regularly but found this quite difficult, as he did not know who I was and was unable to communicate with me.

His condition continued to deteriorate until in July 1999 he had a stroke, which left him bed ridden, and sadly he died on 9 September 1999.

Postscript

I was very sad to have lost my dad but was relieved because it was all over, he no longer had to suffer and I no longer had to watch him suffer.

Having lived with Alzheimer's, I would say that it is a devastating illness. In many ways it affects the carers more, as they are constantly aware of what is happening. It is very hard to watch someone you love slowly lose the ability to live. Alzheimer's patients die long before their actual death. The person you love has gone but their body is still there.

COMMENTARY –
PATSY WESTCOTT

I remember my mother in the summer of 1958 when I was eight years old and she was thirty-eight. We have stopped the car to feed some ducks *en route* to a caravan holiday in Wales. My mother is dark, curly haired, laughing, lighthearted. Later that year she had the first of a series of what were described as nervous breakdowns and darkness descended. I didn't know what a nervous breakdown was, only that my mother had become very odd. She said the assistants in the local Co-op were talking about her. She smelt a strange odour emanating from the coke stove in the corner: my father, she said, was trying to poison her. She wandered into the garden and accosted passing strangers with the question, could they smell the poisonous fumes? Finally – although I only learnt this after he died – she attacked my father with the bread knife. After this she disappeared one day while I was at school. I was told she had been taken to Middlewood, a Victorian mental asylum about twenty miles from where we lived. No one explained why she was there and we (my sister aged three and I) were not allowed to visit. I envisaged her locked in a cross between a prison and Mr Rochester's house in *Jane Eyre*. My father was preoccupied and uncommunicative. When I crept downstairs one night in tears I found him sobbing in the armchair. He seemed embarrassed to be caught thus and brusquely ordered me back to bed. I felt alone and adrift with only the glimmerings of some kind of logic as comfort.

For a week or so while my mother was in the 'loony bin', as it was known, we were looked after by a succession of 'aunties' and home helps. Then an aunt we barely knew (in fact my real aunt, my mother's sister) appeared and whisked my sister and me off to London where she lived. I felt homesick and out of place at my new school, so different from my own cosy, progressive little primary school where we learnt through play and sat at tables. I was teased mercilessly for my northern accent.

No one talked about my mother and my aunt discouraged questions. However, one day, perhaps a month later (the timescale is somewhat hazy), she reappeared with my father, bearing candy babies in sugar-spun lace cradles, seemingly her old self, and we went back home.

Except, everything was different. My mother had had something she called 'shock treatment', which involved strapping her to a table and passing great volts of electricity through her. She complained constantly that it had robbed her of her memory and indeed she seemed to have lost tracts of our shared past. Around this time I saw the film *A Nun's Story* starring Audrey Hepburn with its scene of a 'mad nun' being forced into a strait-jacket. This was what I imagined had happened to my mother.

When I was thirteen my mother suffered a second nervous breakdown. Some playground gossip I had relayed had seemed to trigger the memory of her previous delusions about my father. When my father asked me what I had said and I told him he rounded on me. For years I believed that it was my fault that she had 'broken down'. She was treated locally this time and we weren't sent away. It was less traumatic but still nothing was explained.

Throughout my teens my mother was buried in a quicksand of depression, which stole her energy and *joie de vivre*. She also suffered attacks of acute anxiety she called 'the willies'. She was treated with tranquillisers. She wrote exquisite children's stories…and dark poems, full of foreboding Gothic imagery. She rarely went out. My father did the weekly shopping, while my sister or I shopped locally for daily bread and meat. She wouldn't come to parent–teacher evenings and rarely socialised.

My father's works dinner was an annual ordeal: she was acutely self-conscious and nervous and felt that people viewed her as 'mad'. Her delusions about my father, which she regaled me with whenever she got the chance, continued. She wanted to leave him and they argued. On one occasion she took against one of my friends and forbade me to see her. I felt desperately alone with no one to talk to and became rebellious. I spent as much time as I could out or at friends' houses.

My relationship with my mother was stormy. I was her confidante. I loved, pitied and hated her. There was no one to explain why she behaved as she did or what was wrong.

When I was eighteen I left home to go to university. That year my mother had another breakdown during which she developed delusions about my sister's dance teacher. She was sectioned after a dramatic ambulance chase, which ended with her being bundled, breadknife in hand, into a strait-jacket at the local bus stop: shades of the mad nun. This was a very public humiliation. I was glad I no longer lived at home.

I visited my mother in a psychiatric ward in the local hospital. She seemed calmer, happier, less hostile. For the first time we talked openly about her illness. She told me she had been diagnosed with schizophrenia. She wanted to know more and looked to me 'her clever daughter' to explain.

I had only the vaguest idea what it was.

My mother died when I was twenty-one, of breast cancer. She had had yet another breakdown for which she was treated with drugs, which she told me she would now be on for the rest of her life. For the first time since that far off day on the Welsh borders she seemed happy. At my mother's funeral most of our relatives were unaware that she had been mentally ill. My father and mother had hugged it to themselves, ashamed.

Reading Nicola's report of her experience of her stepfather's mental illness I see that, thirty years on, some things have changed: respite care, day centres, carers, young carers projects, counselling and young carers connection groups were all unknown in the 1960s. Some of Nicola's experiences, however, still find a mirror in my own: her confusion, her feelings of helplessness, the lack of explanation, the assumption that she wouldn't understand.

The last afternoon I spent with my mother before she became terminally ill we went into town. She bought a fur pom-pom hat on a girlish whim. Ironically, to my sister and I, this new 'well' person seemed most unlike our mother. We couldn't get used to her light heartedness. Like Nicola, when she died I felt relieved – almost.

Even today I feel confused when I think about my mother's mental illness. After her death my sister met a psychiatrist who had treated her. He described her as 'one of the worst cases of paranoid schizophrenia' he had ever encountered. Is this true? I still don't know.

Extract from *A Mother's Story*

Georgie Wakefield

Desperate Phone Calls

Desperate phone calls and you're frantic again,
You run on and you're in so much pain,
You're convinced that the nurses are talking about you,
I try to explain that it just isn't true,
I tell you how much they care for you,
But hard as I try it doesn't get through,
Don't leave me here mum, let me come home,
Can you hear them saying things over the phone?
Paul and Sid are bad they do it too,
How on earth can I help you see it's not true?
Remember last Sunday Chris, you accused me of the same,
Then how can I hear them saying my name?
I know that it is pointless when you start to cry,
Saying listen to me mum, you know I don't lie,
I'm not sleeping well, I keep pacing the floor
Please come and get me, I can't take much more,
Mum why's this world so cruel to me?
How do I reply? Can YOU tell me?
Go and speak to the staff Chris, they'll listen to you,
I don't see the point mum, be honest, do you?
I put the phone down, knowing you are still in pain,
Desperate phone calls again and again,
I'll speak to your nurse,
Who will say with a frown,
Just refer him to us and put the phone down,
Feel like running away with nowhere to run,
It's not quite that easy when it's your son.

We'd been down to Dorset I recall
A tragedy we went at all.
13 people hell for you, a terrible mistake I knew
You barely ate or slept at all
Gradually climbing up the wall
Your eyes dart round from one to another
From cousin to auntie from father to mother
Let's go home son, it's best not to stay
No mum, you needed this holiday.
At last we're home, what a relief
But what happened next was beyond belief
We start to unpack, you're looking so sad
"Mum do you think I'm going Mad?"
"I just saw a monster out there in the hall"
No son I don't think you're mad at all
"I could see the saliva between its teeth"
"I was so terrified I shook like a leaf"
The monster your illness showing itself
But you're clearly unwell so I'll get you some help
So I rang my GP for some more medication
Hoping it wouldn't cause too much sedation
Shouldn't do said the doctor just calm him down
Just leave him quiet I'm sure he'll come round
I hear you calling me from your bed
Mum something's wrong with my head
Your head was grotesquely turned around
Your right foot was suspended away from the group
God what's happening to our lad
I'll ring the GP – Steve go tell your dad
Another GP he sounds harassed
Give him 2 procyclidine help at long last
½ hour later and things are worse
God how I hate this evil curse
Rang my GP again at 11.30
Dr arrives and acts quite shirty
Come on you lot get it together

It's so obvious we're at the end of the tether
Such sweet compassion still can't take it in
Can he not see the state we are in?
Get him in your car you'll need A&E
They'll zap him and that will set it free
Paul drives a bit recklessly smokes a cigar
Christian is frantic to get out of the car
Mum he's trying to get out of the door
We're almost there Steve – can we take anymore?
At last the injection you don't make a sound
The nurse pats your bum he's soon come around
We wait 30 minutes the dystonia goes
Sadly and silently make our way home
We're home about 1 (am) and straight to bed
Too shocked to speak so nothing is said
We must put this behind us and look to tomorrow
A trip to dystonia and too much sorrow.

Sleep, Sleep Endless Sleep

Sleep, sleep endless sleep,
Sometimes too lightly sometimes too deep
Hours and hours of every new day
In a darkened room and out of the way,
Sleep endless sleep saps your precious time,
It makes no difference if the weather is fine,
At a time when life should be free from care,
I should call you once more but I don't think I dare,
You will only get angry and say go away,
Sleep endless sleep steals another new day,
You rise about five I make you some tea,
I say what a waste you say yes I agree,
You're ready for bed by 10pm,
It seems that you're ready to sleep yet again,
Sleep endless sleep, and I pray that tomorrow,
You may get up early, and stop all of this sorrow,
I've prayed for years though god knows why,
Sometimes I question if you really try,
Sleep endless sleep, and I can't understand
Why you need all this sleep when you're such a young man,
One day you'll wake out of bed you will leap,
Full of life, no more endless sleep,
Full of zest and facing a full young life,
Free from fatigue, sadness and strife,
This is a dream in my soul I'll keep,
That the day will come you won't need endless sleep.

GLOSSARY OF TERMS

ORGANISATIONS THAT CAN HELP

REFERENCES AND RECOMMENDED READING

INDEX

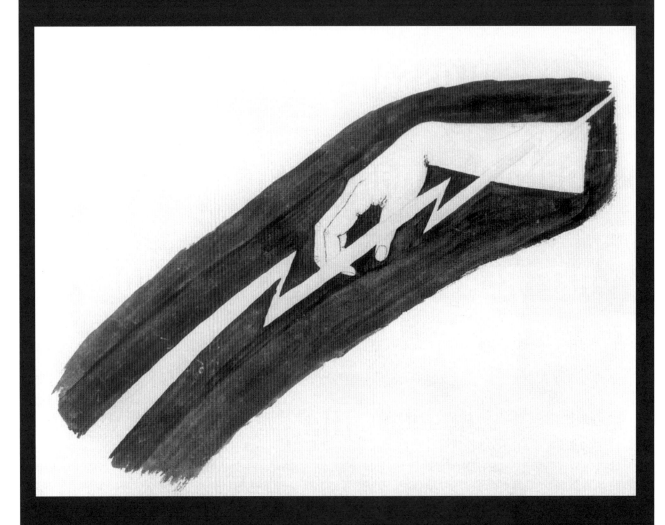

From the Adamson Collection

GLOSSARY OF TERMS

Alzheimer's (disease): a progressive illness affecting the brain and causing dementia, primarily in the elderly.

Anorexia nervosa: an eating disorder involving an intense fear of fatness, under eating and excessive loss of weight.

Bipolar (affective) disorder: a mood disorder in which both manic and depressive episodes occur.

Bulimia: a serious eating disorder characterised by a fear of fatness, binge-eating, vomiting and excessive use of laxatives.

Chronic (mentally ill): a term for patients with severe mental illness who need continuing care for long periods and different levels of intensity depending on their needs and response to treatment. Also of a disease, deep seated or long continued (as opposed to acute).

Cocaine: a drug obtained from coca leaves or produced synthetically. It is a powerful stimulant that produces a sense of exhilaration and reduced fatigue and hunger.

Counselling: a general term that is used to cover several processes of interviewing, testing, guiding, advising and so on, to help, for example, an individual solve problems or plan the future.

Delirium: the state of being 'delirious', which is the wandering of the mind, especially through fever or other illness; wild excitement.

Dementia: a disorder that causes serious memory problems. The commonest is Alzheimer's disease.

Detoxification (detox): the process of withdrawing a person from an addictive substance in a safe and effective way.

Diagnosis: the identification of a disease by means of its symptoms.

Electroconvulsive therapy (ECT): a physical treatment for severe depressive illness. During ECT a small amount of electric current is passed across the brain for usually two to three seconds. This produces an artificial epileptic fit. ECT is only given under a general aneasthetic.

Epilepsy: a chronic functional disease of the nervous system with recurring attacks of sudden unconsciousness, accompanied by convulsive seizures.

Forensic psychiatrist (legal psychiatrist): a psychiatrist who is concerned with people with mental illness who break the law. They work in a variety of places, which can include special hospitals (such as Broadmoor) and prisons.

GP: general practitioner or family doctor.

Hallucination: happens when you hear, smell, feel or see something when there isn't anything, or anybody, actually there to hear, smell, feel or see. In schizophrenia the commonest hallucination is hearing voices.

Hypomania: less intensive form of **mania**, which is characterised by (a) an elated or irritable mood; (b) increased physical activity, restlessness and agitation; and (c) an increase in the number of ideas or in the speed of thinking and speaking.

Insomnia: sleeplessness; a chronic inability to obtain the amount of sleep necessary to maintain adequate daytime behaviour.

Maladaptive: faulty adaptation.

Malignant: disposed to do harm; tending to cause death, spreading or deteriorating rapidly, especially of a tumour or cancer.

Marijuana: another word for cannabis.

Menopause: ending of menstruation, change of life.

Mortality: frequency or number of deaths in proportion to the population.

Obsessive–compulsive disorder (OCD): a form of anxiety disorder that is characterised by recurrent, disturbing, unwanted intrusive thoughts, or repetitive actions.

Paranoia: a form of mental disorder characterised by constant delusions, especially of grandeur, pride, persecution; intense, and often irrational, fear or suspicion.

Pharmacology: the science of drugs.

Phobia: an anxiety disorder consisting of an irrational and morbid fear of an object or situation.

Psychiatrist: a medically qualified doctor who deals with the prevention, diagnosis and treatment of mental and emotional disorders.

Psychoanalysis: a method of investigation and psychotherapy whereby psychological difficulties are traced to forgotten hidden concepts in the patient's mind and treated by bringing them to light.

Psychoses: showing the signs or having the characteristics of severe mental disorder.

Psychotherapy: there are many different types of psychotherapy. They are all ways of helping people to overcome stress, emotional problems, relationship problems or troublesome habits. Treatment is based on talking to another person and sometimes doing things together.

Rehabilitation: a programme of treatment and re-adjustment to life to prepare the person with mental illness physically, mentally, socially and vocationally for the fullest possible life.

Schizophrenia: a mental illness that affects about one out of every hundred people. There are many popular myths and misunderstanding about it and it does not mean a 'split personality'. People who suffer from schizophrenia experience 'positive' symptoms such as hallucinations or delusions or muddled thinking and 'negative' symptoms, which means that your interest in life, energy, emotions and 'get-up-and-go' just drain away.

Speed: slang word for amphetamines, which are synthetic and potentially habit-forming drugs that stimulate the central nervous system.

Stigma: is a mark of disgrace or infamy. In the context of mental disorders, it means being discriminated against by others through prejudice, ignorance and fear.

Therapeutic: relating to the curing of disease; contributing towards or performed to improve health or general well-being.

Trauma: injury, damage, wound or shock.

ORGANISATIONS THAT CAN HELP

This information is as up-to-date as possible when going to print.

Alcohol Concern	Waterbridge House, 32–36 Loman Street, London SE1 0EE Tel: 020 7992 8667 (1–5pm, Mon–Fri) Drinkline: 0800 917 8282 (equivalent of a helpline) E-mail: info@alcoholconcern.org.uk http://www.alcoholconcern.org.uk
Alzheimer's Society	Gordon House, 10 Greencoat Place, London SW1P 1PH Tel: 020 7306 0606 Fax: 020 7306 0808 http://www.alzheimers.org.uk
Association of Post-Natal Illness	25 Jerdan Place, Fulham, London SW6 1BE Tel: 020 7386 0868
BTSTEPS **(Telephone-based system of** **behavioural therapy for OCD)**	Operates from the NHS Stress Self-Help Clinic 303 North End Road, London W14 9NS Tel: 020 7610 2594 http://www.fearfighter.com/frontpage/nhs_stress_self.htm
Carers UK	20–25 Glasshouse Yard, London EC1A 4TJ Tel: 020 7490 8818 Carer's line: 0808 808 7777 (10am–12noon and 2–4pm, Mon–Fri) Fax: 020 7490 8824 http://www.carersonline.org.uk
Changing Minds	C/o The Royal College of Psychiatrists 17 Belgrave Square, London SW1X 8PG Tel: 020 7235 2351 Fax: 020 7245 1231 http://www.rcpsych.ac.uk/campaigns/cminds/index.htm

CRUSE Bereavement Care	Cruse House, 126 Sheen Road, Richmond, Surrey TW9 1UR Tel: 020 8939 9530 Helpline: 0870 167 1677 (9.30am–5.00pm, Mon–Fri) Fax: 020 8940 7638 E-mail: info@crusebereavementcare.org.uk
Depression Alliance	35 Westminster Bridge Road, London SE1 7JB Tel: 0207 633 0557 Fax: 020 7633 0559 http://www.depressionalliance.org
DrugScope	32–36 Loman Street, London SE1 0EE Tel: 020 7928 1211 Fax: 020 7928 1771 http://www.drugscope.org.uk
Eating Disorders Association	103 Prince of Wales Road, Norwich NR1 1DW Adult helpline: 0845 634 1414 (8.30am–8.30pm, Mon–Fri) Youthline: 0845 634 7650 (open 4.00–6.30pm, weekdays)
Manic Depression Fellowship	Castle Works, 21 St George's Road, London SE1 6ES Tel: 020 7793 2600 Fax: 020 7793 2639 E-mail: mdf@mdf.org.uk http://www.mdf.org.uk
Medical Foundation for the Care of Victims of Torture	96–98 Grafton Road, Kentish Town, London NW5 3EJ Tel: 020 7813 7777 Fax: 020 7813 0011 E-mail: clinical@torturecare.org.uk http://www.torturecare.org.uk
Mental Health Foundation	UK Office: 7th Floor, 83 Victoria Street, London SW1H 0HW Tel: 020 7802 0300

	Fax: 020 7802 0301
	E-mail: mhf@mhf.org.uk
	http://www.mentalhealth.org.uk
Mind	Granta House, 15–19 Broadway, London E15 4BQ
	Tel: 020 8519 2122
	MindinfoLine: 08457 660 163 (9.15am–5.15pm, Mon–Fri)
	Fax: 020 8522 1725
	E-mail: contact@mind.org.uk
	http://www.mind.org.uk
NAFSIYAT **Inter Cultural Therapy Centre**	278 Seven Sisters Road, Finsbury Park, London N1 2HY Tel: 020 7263 4130
National Family and **Parenting Institute**	430 Highgate Studios, 53–79 Highgate Road, London NW5 1TL
	Tel: 020 7424 3460
	Fax: 020 7485 3590
	E-mail: info@nfpi.org
	http://www.nfpi.org
National Phobics Society	Zion Community Resource Centre, 339 Stretford Road, Hulme, Manchester M15 4ZY
	Tel: 0870 7700 456
	Fax: 0161 227 9862
	http://www.phobics-society.org.uk
National Schizophrenia Fellowship **New working name: Rethink**	Head Office, 30 Tabernacle Street, London EC2A 4DD
	Tel: 020 7330 9100/01
	National advice line: 020 8974 6814 (10am–3pm, Mon–Fri)
	Fax: 020 7330 9102
	http://www.nsf.org.uk
NHS Direct **(24-hour nurse-led helpline)**	Tel: 0845 4647 http://www.nhsdirect.nhs.uk

Relate	Herbert Gray College, Little Church Street, Rugby, Warwickshire CV21 3AP Tel: 01788 573 241 Fax: 01788 535 007 http://www.relate.org.uk
SANE	1st Floor, Cityside House, 40 Adler Street, London E1 1EE Tel: 020 7375 1002 Helpline: 0845 767 8000 (12noon–2am) Fax: 020 7375 2162 http://www.sane.org.uk
The Samaritans	The Samaritans, The Upper Mill, Kingston Road, Ewell, Surrey KT17 2AF Tel: 020 8394 8300 Helpline: 08457 90 90 90 Fax: 020 8394 8301 E-mail: admin@samaritans.org http://www.samaritans.co.uk
The Traumatic Stress Clinic	73 Charlotte Street, London W1T 4PL Tel: 020 7530 3666 Fax: 020 7530 3677 http://www.uktrauma.org.uk
Triumph Over Phobia	PO Box 1831, Bath BA2 4YW Tel: 01225 330353 Fax: 01225 469212 http://www.triumphoverphobia.com
Turning Point (Social care organisation)	New Loom House, 101 Backchurch Lane, London E1 1LU Tel: 020 7553 5500 E-mail: info@turning-point.co.uk http://www.turning-point.co.uk
Young Minds	102–108 Clerkenwell Road, London EC1M 5SA Tel: 020 7336 8445 YoungMinds Parents' Information Service: 0800 018 2138 Fax: 020 7336 8446 http://www.youngminds.org.uk

REFERENCES AND RECOMMENDED READING

Aldridge, S. (2000) *Seeing Red and Feeling Blue*. London: Century.

Andrew Watkiss v John Laing plc (2000) Jilly Welsh Mental Block. *People Management*, 20 January.

Cobb, A. (2000) *Mind Guide to Surviving Working Life*. London: Mind.

Coleman, J. (2001) Understanding self-esteem. *YoungMinds Magazine*, **51**, 18–19.

Conrad, J. (1900) *Lord Jim*. London: Pan Books.

Copeland, M. E. (1992) *The Depression Workbook. A Guide to Living with Depression and Manic Depression*. Oakland, CA: New Harbinger Publishers.

Crowe, M. & Bunclark, J. (2000) Repeated self-injury and its management. *International Review of Psychiatry*, **12**, 48–53.

—— & Dare, C. (1998) Survivors of childhood sexual abuse: approaches to therapy. *Advances in Psychiatric Treatment*, **4**, 96–100.

Dunn, S. & Crawford, L. (1999) *Creating Accepting Communities: Report of the Mind Inquiry into Social Exclusion and Mental Health Problems*. London: Mind.

EDA (2000*a*) *Eating Disorders in the U.K. Review of the Provision of Health Care Services for Men with Eating Disorders*. Norwich: EDA.

—— (2000*b*) *Men with Eating Disorders - The Hidden Minority?* (Press Release 14-2-00). London: EDA.

Employers' Forum on Disability (1998) *A Practical Guide to Employment Adjustments for People with Mental Health Problems*. Briefing Guide 5. London: Employers' Forum on Disability.

Ferguson, S. (1973) *A Guard Within*. London: Chatto & Windus.

Foskett, J. H. (1999) Soul searching within the service. *Mental Health, Religion and Culture*, **2**, 11–17.

Frame, J. (1961) *Faces in the Water*. London: Women's Press.

Glozier, N. (1998) Workplace effects of the stigmatization of depression. *Journal of Occupational and Environmental Medicine*, **40**, 793–800.

Gowers, S. G. (2000) Eating Disorders. In *Adolescent Psychiatry in Clinical Practice*, pp 211–230. London: Edward Arnold Publishers.

Health Education Authority(1999) *Promoting Mental Health. The Role of Faith Communities: Jewish and Christian Perspectives*. London: Health Education Authority.

Linehan, M. M. (1993) *Cognitive-Behavioural Treatment of Borderline Personality Disorder*. New York: Guildford Press.

Lott, T. (1996) *The Scent of Dried Roses*. London: Viking.

Mental Health Foundation (1997) *Knowing our Own Minds*. London: Mental Health Foundation.

Millett, K. (1991) *The Loony-bin Trip*. London: Virago.

Milligan, S. & Clare, A. (1995) *Depression and How to Survive It*. London: Ebury Press.

Mind (2000) *Surviving Working Life: The Mind Guide to Staying Well in the Workplace*. London: Mind.

—— (2000) *Managing for Mental Health: the Mind Employers' Resource Pack*. London: Mind.

Neeleman, J. & King, M. B. (1993) Psychiatrists' religious attitudes in relation to their clinical practice. *Acta Psychiatrica Scandanavica*, **88**, 420–424.

Perry, A., Tarrier, N., Morriss, R., *et al* (1999) Randomised controlled trial of efficacy of teaching patients with bipolar disorder to identify early symptoms of relapse and obtain treatment. *BMJ*, **318**, 149–153.

Plath, S. (1963) *The Bell Jar*. London: William Heinemann.

Rooke-Matthews, S. & Lindow, V. (1998) *Survivors Guide to Working in the Mental Health Services*. London: Mind.

Rutter, M. & Smith, D. J. (1995) *Psychosocial Disorders in Young People: Times, Trends and their Courses*. Chichester: John Wiley.

Sainsbury Centre for Mental Health (1998) *Acute Problems: A Survey of the Quality of Care in Acute Psychiatric Wards*. London: Sainsbury Centre for Mental Health.

Salkovskis, P. M., Atha, C. & Storer, D. (1990) Cognitive-behavioural problem solving in the treatment of patients who repeatedly attempt suicide. A controlled trial. *British Journal of Psychiatry*, **157**, 871–876.

Schreber, D. (1903) *Memoirs of my Nervous Illness* (trans. I. Macalpine & R. Hunter). London: Dawson & Sons.

Shaw, F. (1997) *Out of Me*. London: Viking.

Stephenson, R. L. (1886) *Strange Case of Dr Jekyll and Mr Hyde*. London: Longmans, Green and Co.

Styron, W. (1991) *Darkness Visible*. London: Jonathan Cape.

Summerfield, D. (1999) A critique of seven assumptions behind psychological trauma programmes in war-affected areas. *Social Science & Medicine*, **48**, 1449–1462.

—— (2001) Asylum-seekers, refugees and mental health services in the UK. *Psychiatric Bulletin*, **25**, 161–163.

Szasz, T. (1988) *The Myth of Psychotherapy. Mental Healing as Religion, Rhetoric, and Repression*. Syracuse, NY: Syracuse University Press.

Tufnell, G. (ed) (1999) *Mental Health and Growing Up*. Factsheets. London: Royal College of Psychiatrists.

Wolpert, L. (1999) *Malignant Sadness: The Anatomy of Depression*. London: Faber & Faber.

Zarowsky, C. (2000) Trauma stories: violence, emotion and politics in Somali Ethopia. *Transcultural Psychiatry,* **37**, 383–402.

INDEX

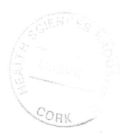